Intelligent Systems in Healthcare and Disease Identification using Data Science

The health technology has become a hot topic in academic research. It employs the theory of social networks into the different levels of the prediction and analysis and has brought new possibilities for the development of technology. This book is a descriptive summary of challenges and methods using disease identification with various case studies from diverse authors across the globe.

One of the new buzzwords in healthcare sector that has become popular over years is health informatics. Healthcare professionals must deal with an increasing number of computers and computer programs in their daily work. With rapid growth of digital data, the role of analytics in healthcare has created a significant impact on healthcare professional's life. Improvements in storage data, computational power and parallelization has also contributed to uptake this technology. This book is intended for use by researchers, health informatics professionals, academicians and undergraduate and postgraduate students interested in knowing more about health informatics. It aims to provide a brief overview about informatics, its history and area of practice, laws in health informatics, challenges and technologies in health informatics, application of informatics in various sectors and so on. Finally, the research avenues in health informatics along with some case studies are discussed.

Intelligent Systems in Healthcare and Disease Identification using Data Science

Edited by
Gururaj H L, Radhika A D
Divya C D, Ravi Kumar V
and Yu-Chen Hu

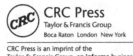

CRC Press
Taylor & Francis Group
Boca Raton London New York

CRC Press is an imprint of the
Taylor & Francis Group, an **informa** business

A CHAPMAN & HALL BOOK

Designed cover image: PopTika/Shutterstock

First edition published 2024
by CRC Press
2385 NW Executive Center Dr. Suite 320, Boca Raton, FL 33431

and by CRC Press
4 Park Square, Milton Park, Abingdon, Oxon, OX14 4RN

CRC Press is an imprint of Taylor & Francis Group, LLC

© 2024 selection and editorial matter, Gururaj H L, Radhika A D, Divya C D, Ravi Kumar V, Yu-Chen Hu; individual chapters, the contributors

Reasonable efforts have been made to publish reliable data and information, but the author and publisher cannot assume responsibility for the validity of all materials or the consequences of their use. The authors and publishers have attempted to trace the copyright holders of all material reproduced in this publication and apologize to copyright holders if permission to publish in this form has not been obtained. If any copyright material has not been acknowledged please write and let us know so we may rectify in any future reprint.

Except as permitted under U.S. Copyright Law, no part of this book may be reprinted, reproduced, transmitted, or utilized in any form by any electronic, mechanical, or other means, now known or hereafter invented, including photocopying, microfilming, and recording, or in any information storage or retrieval system, without written permission from the publishers.

For permission to photocopy or use material electronically from this work, access www.copyright.com or contact the Copyright Clearance Center, Inc. (CCC), 222 Rosewood Drive, Danvers, MA 01923, 978-750-8400. For works that are not available on CCC please contact mpkbookspermissions@tandf.co.uk

Trademark notice: Product or corporate names may be trademarks or registered trademarks and are used only for identification and explanation without intent to infringe.

ISBN: 9781032406633 (hbk)
ISBN: 9781032406657 (pbk)
ISBN: 9781003354178 (ebk)

DOI: 10.1201/9781003354178

Typeset in Times
by Newgen Publishing UK

Contents

Preface vii
Editor Bio ix
List of Contributors xi

Chapter 1   Basics of Healthcare Informatics 1
                 J. Sudeep, M. Goutham, G. Prasannakumar, K. Raghavendra and S. C. Girish

Chapter 2   Foundation of Medical Data Sciences 35
                 S. M. Bramesh

Chapter 3   Fundamentals and Technicalities of Big Data and Analytics 51
                 Partha Ghosh, Ananya Biswas and Suradhuni Ghosh

Chapter 4   Fundamentals of Health Informatics and Health Data Science 107
                 N. S. Prema

Chapter 5   Introduction to Disease Prediction 121
                 K. V. H. Avani, Deeksha Manjunath and C. Gururaj

Chapter 6   Medical Record Management for Disease Management 189
                 Gururaj H. L., Soundarya Bidare Chandre Gowda and D. Basavesha

Chapter 7   Prediction Models for Health Care 209
                 Kiran, M. S. Hemanth Kumar, D. S. Sunil Kumar, M. T. Ganesh Kumar and S. Nandini

Chapter 8   Application of Image Processing in the Detection of Plant Diseases 225
                 Pawan Whig, Nasmin Jiwani, Ketan Gupta, Shama Kouser, Arun Velu and Ashima Bhatia

Chapter 9 Preprocessing Sparse and Commonly Evolving
Standardised Health Records 243

*C. D. Divya, A. B. Rajendra, and
Soundarya Bidare Chandre Gowda*

Chapter 10 A Decision-Making System for Clinical Data 259

*Natarajan Rajesh, M. Natesh, Anitha Premkumar,
V. Karthik and T. Ramesh*

Index 277

Preface

This book is a descriptive summary of the challenges and methods used in disease identification with various case studies from diverse authors across the globe.

The authors of Chapter1 elaborate the fundamentals of health informatics using two categories of health, mental and physical health. Balanced diet, regular exercises and adequate amount of rest will contribute to good health. An individual with good corporeal health is expected to have optimal function and process the work at peak. Mental fitness is as important as that of physical fitness, which relates to social, emotional and psychological well-being of an individual.

In Chapter 2, the authors discuss the different clinical datasets and techniques along with their advantages and disadvantages for mining comorbidity patterns in patients with diabetes. This chapter will serve as a primer for researchers to assimilate the use of electronic health records (EHRs) in gaining insights into comorbidity patterns in patients with diabetes.

The authors of Chapters 3 and 4 provide an overview of definition, characteristics, types, components, benefits, analytical tools and technologies, and most recent insights. A case study demonstrates the importance of disease identification and diagnosis. Big data can be used to improve the healthcare systems.

The authors of Chapters 5 and 6 are concerned with the need for user-friendly software, appropriate training on using EHR and robust and fast network connectivity to allow quick access to the patient's prior information as well as speedy record storing. Making the use of EHRs mandatory in all the health centres will speed up the transition from manual to electronic health records systems and may even result in interoperability.

The authors of Chapters 7 and 8 use the CNN architecture algorithms on image processing and requisition of the desire portion from MR images. Furthermore, we used different machine learning algorithms (kernel SVM, KNN) for the detection of brain tumour.

The authors of Chapters 9 and 10 focus on training data propagation that can be evenly distributed by using a synthetic minority oversampling (SMOTE-Out) technique. Heart disease can be predicted using the proposed WFRNN, which incorporates the GA. The stat log dataset was employed in this study. The proposed model scored better than those of existing models and earlier studies.

H. L. Gururaj

Editor Bio

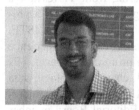

H. L. Gururaj is currently working as Associate Professor, Department of Information Technology, Manipal Institute of Technology, Bengaluru, India. He holds a PhD degree in Computer Science and Engineering from Visvesvaraya Technological University, Belagavi, India. He is a professional member of ACM and works as ACM Distinguished Speaker. He is the founder of Wireless Internetworking Group (WiNG). He is a senior member of IEEE and lifetime member of ISTE and CSI. He has received a young scientist award from the Government of India. He has eight years of teaching experience at both the undergraduate and postgraduate level. His research interests include block chain technology, cyber security, wireless sensor network, ad-hoc networks, IOT, data mining, cloud computing and machine learning. He has guided 30 undergraduate students and 10 postgraduate students. He is an Editorial Board member of the *International Journal of Block Chains and Cryptocurrencies* (IJBC) and editor of EAI publishers. He has published more than 75 research papers including two ESCI publications in various international journals such in Science Citation Index, IEEE Access, Springer Book Chapter, Scopus, and UGC refereed journals. He has presented 20 papers at various international conferences. He has authored one book on network simulators. He worked as a reviewer for various journals and conferences.

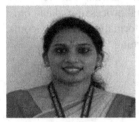

A. D. Radhika has completed her M. Tech in Computer Science and Engineering from Visvesvaraya Technological University. She was working as Assistant Professor in the Department of Computer Science and Engineering at Vidyavardhaka College of Engineering Mysore, Karnataka. She is pursuing her PhD from Visvesvaraya Technological University. She has published nine research papers in various reputed international journals and conferences. Her areas of interest include artificial intelligence, data science, machine learning, and image processing.

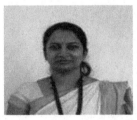

C. D. Divya has completed M. Tech her in Computer Science and Engineering from Visvesvaraya Technological University. She is currently working as Assistant Professor in the Department of Computer Science and Engineering at Vidyavardhaka College of Engineering, Mysore, Karnataka. She is pursuing her PhD from Visvesvaraya Technological University. She has published 15 research papers in various reputed international journals and conferences. Her areas of interest include artificial intelligence, data science, machine learning, and image processing. She worked as reviewer for various journals and conferences.

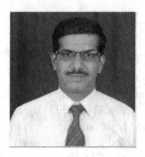

V. Ravi Kumar is currently working as Dean in the Faculty of Computer Sciences, Vidyavardhaka College of Engineering, Mysuru, India. He received his PhD in Computer Science and Engineering from Visvesvaraya Technological University, Belagavi, India. He is a professional member of ACM and lifetime member of ISTE, IETE, and CSI. He has 16 years of teaching experience at both the undergraduate and postgraduate level. His research interests include block chain technology, data mining and machine learning. He has guided 50 undergraduate students and 18 postgraduate students. He is an Editorial Board member of the *International Journal of Block Chains and Cryptocurrencies* (IJBC). He has published more than 52 research papers including two ESCI publications in various international journals such in Science Citation Index, IEEE Access, Springer Book Chapter, Scopus, and UGC refereed journals. He has presented 20 papers at various international conferences. He worked as reviewer for various journals and conferences.

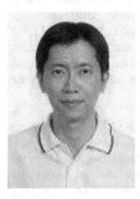

Yu-Chen Hu received his PhD in computer science and information engineering from the Department of Computer Science and Information Engineering, National Chung Cheng University, Chiayi, Taiwan in 1999. Currently, Dr. Hu is a professor in the Department of Computer Science and Information Management, Providence University, Sha-Lu, Taiwan. His research interests include image and signal processing, data compression, information hiding, information security, computer network, and machine learning.

Contributors

Avani, K. V. H.
B.M.S. College of Engineering, Bengaluru

Basavesha, D.
Shridevi Institute of Engineering and Technology, Tumkur

Bhatia, Ashima
Vivekananda Institute of Professional Studies, New Delhi

Biswas, Ananya
Govt. College of Engineering and Ceramic Technology, Kolkata

Bramesh, S. M.
PES, Mandya

Divya, C. D.
Vidyavardhaka College of Engineering, Mysuru, India

Ganesh Kumar, M. T.
G. Madegowda Institute of Technology, Mandya, Karnataka, India

Ghosh, Partha
Govt. College of Engineering and Ceramic Technology, Kolkata

Ghosh, Suradhuni
Govt. Girls' General Degree College, Ekbalpur, Kolkata

Girish, S. C.
The National Institute of Engineering (North Campus), Mysuru, Karnataka, India

Goutham, M.
Dayanand Sagar University, Bengaluru, Karnataka, India

Gowda, Soundarya Bidare Chandre
Alva's Institute of Engineering and Technology, Mangalore, India

Gupta, Ketan
University of The Cumberlands, USA

Gururaj, C.
B.M.S. College of Engineering, Bengaluru

Gururaj, H. L.
Manipal Institute of Technology Bengaluru

Hemanth Kumar, M. S.
G. Madegowda Institute of Technology, Mandya, Karnataka, India

Shama, Kouser
University, Saudi Arabia

Jiwani, Nasmin
University of The Cumberlands, USA

Karthik, V.
M. S. Ramaiah institute of technology, Bangalore, India

Kiran
Vidyavardhaka College of Engineering, Mysuru, Karnataka, India

Kumar, Sumit
Tata Main Hospital, India

Manjunath, Deeksha
B.M.S. College of Engineering,
 Bengaluru

Nandini, S.
Kalpataru Institute of Technology,
 Tiptur, Karnataka, India

Natesh, M.
Vidyavardhaka College of Engineering,
 Mysuru, India

Prasannakumar, G.
The National Institute of Engineering
 (North Campus), Mysuru,
 Karnataka, India

Prema, N. S.
Vidyavardhaka College of
 Engineering, Mysuru

Premkumar, Anitha
Presidency University, Bangalore, India

Raghavendra, K.
The National Institute of Engineering
 (North Campus), Mysuru,
 Karnataka, India

Rajendra, A. B.
Vidyavardhaka College of Engineering,
 Mysuru, India

Rajesh, Natarajan
University of Technology and Applied
 Sciences-Shinas, Oman

Sudeep, J.
The National Institute of Engineering
 (North Campus), Mysuru,
 Karnataka, India

Ramesh, T.
Presidency University, Bangalore, India

Sunil Kumar, D. S.
Administrative Management College,
 Bangalore, Karnataka, India

Velu, Arun
Equifax, USA

Whig, Pawan
Vivekananda Institute of Professional
 Studies, New Delhi

1 Basics of Healthcare Informatics

J. Sudeep, M. Goutham, G. Prasannakumar, K. Raghavendra and S. C. Girish

1.1 BACKGROUND

The use computers has significantly impacted all sectors of the society. Based on individual needs, computers are designed to serve various purposes. It could be for a general or a specific purpose. The computers designed for general purpose have limited computing capabilities and are used for commercial or any other application. On the other hand, those designed for specific purposes have high processing power and resources that could solve complex manipulations and instructions and thus can be utilized for scientific and military applications.

Informatics is the integration of people, information and technology. Health informatics is regarded as one of the fastest growing scientific disciplines that deals with theory and practice of processing the information in the field of health science employing information and communication technology. The advancement of communication and information technology, on the one hand, and the adoption of these new technologies in healthcare sectors, on the other, have a significant impact on various interdisciplinary domains.

1.2 OVERVIEW OF HEALTH INFORMATICS

The advent of health informatics began during both the World Wars I and II, which awakened the clinicians and researchers that the potential use of computers could aid in diagnosis the health diseases. Over the past 30 years, the rapid developments in information and communication technology (ICT) have given rise to several theories and models in the field of health informatics.

One of the buzzwords in the healthcare sector today is "health informatics." Health informatics is one of the fastest growing fields, which uses computer science and information technology to solve health-related problems. It provides tools for the preparation, acquisition and distribution of medical data. Health informatics uses self-automated routing tasks that involve the development of technology in various diverse fields of engineering. Health informatics should benefit health care professionals in providing better and efficient solutions to solve the needs of the patients. Healthcare professionals capture, communicate and use clinical data and knowledge to support them. There are numerous definitions proposed on health informatics:

> Health Informatics is one such area of engineering sciences which deals with development of methods & technologies for acquisition, processing & study of patient data with scientific knowledge research.

[1]

Health informatics not only provides the solution to solve the health care problems but also covers all aspects of generation, retrieval, analysis and data synthesis to improve healthcare. The primary purpose of health informatics is to provide effective healthcare to the patients.

1.2.1 WHY IS HEALTH INFORMATICS IMPORTANT?

Health informatics has become an integral component of healthcare. The importance of health informatics and the people who work in it has increased significantly in the age of big data. Health informatics is crucial to healthcare industry, although many healthcare professionals work in the background to organize, store and manage health data using electronic health records to improve the patient experience. By utilizing the information and communication technologies, the healthcare professionals will have an easier access to patient information, which allows doctors, nurses and other paramedics to quickly take decisions and achieve efficient results [2].

1.2.2 TYPES OF HEALTH INFORMATICS

Health informatics can be broadly classified into various types:

- Clinical informatics
- Population health informatics
- Medicinal informatics
- Public health informatics
- Consumer health informatics
- Nursing informatics
- Dental informatics
- Nutrition informatics
- Pharmacy informatics
- Pathology informatics
- Biomedical informatics
- Translational bioinformatics
- Computational health informatics
- Clinical research informatics
- Mental health informatics
- Nutrition informatics

- Neuroengineering and neuroinformatics
- Informatics in active and healthy ageing

1.2.3 Domains of Health Information Practice

The field of health informatics is said to be young and dynamic. To continuously improve the design of the system, it is essential to identify the requirements that change over time so that a strong information system in health field can be put in place. This also helps improve the quality of care and empower the health superintendents for decentralized planning and management by giving patients access to more health information. The health informatics subdomains includes human resource management, hospital information system, health management information system, geographical information system and mobile-specific program monitoring system. Figure 1.1 [3] shows the Venn diagram of domains proposed by AMIA Accreditation Committee.

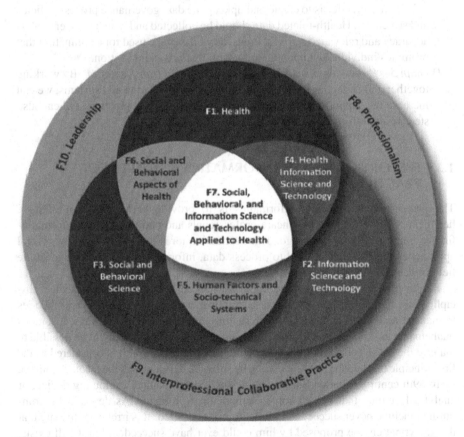

FIGURE 1.1 Venn diagram of domains proposed by AMIA Accreditation Committee [3].

Some of domains of health information practice are listed below:

Domain 1 – Foundational knowledge: The basic skills and knowledge that give health informaticians a shared language, a foundational understanding of all health informatics field and an awareness of environment in which they work.

Domain 2 – Enhanced medical decision-making processes and outcomes: The main goal is to support clinical and public health professionals by examining the current health process to determine how medical data and medical information systems can lead to better outcomes. It assesses the influence of health information system on practice and pursues innovation and discovery in medical information systems and information practice.

Domain 3 – Health Information Systems: Special considerations for security, privacy and safety must be taken into account when planning, developing, acquiring, implementing, maintaining and evaluating the integration of health information system with current information technology systems used throughout the healthcare that includes clinical, consumer and public health domains.

Domain 4 – Analytics and data governance management: Another domain of health informatics practice is to create and upkeep the data governance process policies and structures. Health-related data should be collected and managed to ensure its accuracy and relevance across settings, as well as to be used for examination that promotes individual and population health that drives innovation.

Domain 5 – Professionalism, strategy, leadership and transformation: By working together and engaging stakeholders across the organization and systems, we can increase the support and alignment with informatics best practices and can also steer health informatics efforts and innovation [4].

1.3 HISTORY OF HEALTH INFORMATICS AND AREAS OF PRACTICE

The primary goal of health informatics is to provide better and cost-effective healthcare solutions to the healthcare professionals and patients. Health informatics first emerged nearly 70 years ago. This section explores the earlier roots on several approaches the researchers used to process data, information and knowledge in the field of health informatics.

Health informatics is a young discipline when compared with other medical disciplines. In the 17th century, many researchers attempted to propose several theories to manage real-world problems by representing information in many ways. A famous mathematician Wilhelm Von Leibnitz came up with the idea that it might be possible to manage the entire behaviour of human nature in a codified form. It is considered as the first principle that laid the basis for coding by software developers in the medical domain.

In 19th century, Charles Babbage built the first mechanical computing device, or analytical engine, that helped solve mathematical problems. As desired, the computing machine never succeeded in functioning as desired. It is irrelevant to state that the analytical engine proposed by him could ever have succeeded, but it still exists. There is a debate whether the analytical engine has succeeded or not [5].

The above two examples illustrate that real-life problems can be solved easily if enough accurate engineering techniques are made available.

During World War II, several healthcare providers and researchers examined the possibilities of using computers to aid in disease diagnosis. This eventually led to the introduction of mainframes computers in hospitals at the beginning of the 20th century.

1.3.1 THE EARLY DAYS

In the 1950s, professionals from a variety of fields such as bioengineering, epidemiology, clinical documentation and biophysics started to work together on early projects of health informatics. As a result, the International Society of Cybernetic Drugs was established in 1958. The Cybernetic Senate was held in Naples in 1960 and a new journal showcasing research in health documentation and statistics was launched. This led to the early developments of health informatics.

1.3.2 EVOLUTION OF COMPUTING AND DATA ANALYSIS

The study of computational systems that support the digital data for efficient storage and retrieval operations is called informatics. The first independent organization for informatics was started by Gutsav Wagner in Germany in the year 1949. In the 1950s, it became a distinct discipline and in the 1960s, it was recognized as the separate field of study. Before the term informatics was coined, the field had different names like biomedical computing, medical information science, computer medicine, medical computing and medical information processing that reflected the way the technology was used in the healthcare sector. With the evolution of computer technology, the focus of health informatics was to develop standards for digitizing health records using software and hardware. In the year 1960, significant advancement in the usage of computers helped to perform numerous medical tasks. In 1967, Utah University built the first electronic medical record (EMR) system called HELP (Health Evaluation through Logical Programming). It was launched in Latter-Day Saints Hospital and supported laboratories of pharmacy, radiology and heart care units before getting expanded to a full-fledged laboratory. During the 1970s and mid-1980s, the computers shrank and grew more portable. Laptops and desktop models became practical, which was a useful tool for clinics and hospitals of all sizes. In the year 1970, an independent organization called International Medical Informatics Association (IMIA) was started to promote the use of computers in the domain of healthcare, bioscience and medicine to serve the needs of the society. In 1987, it got transformed into a technical committee, International Federation for Information Processing (IFIP), and became an independent organization. The community of health informatics matured and continues to grow over the years. New programs were introduced in health informatics for data analysis such as patient scheduling and digital order entry system. The federal government funded millions of dollars to Science Application International Corp (SAIC) to build a computerized healthcare system for the Department of Defense [5].

1.3.3 Moving towards Digital Healthcare

The evolution, digitization and promise of technology in healthcare such as medical treatment, information sharing, diagnosis and record keeping was widely acknowledged by healthcare authorities in the early 2000. The rapid adoption of digitized modern devices that supported computerized health records was aimed at avoiding mistakes in medical healthcare so as to reduce the cost and improve the care delivered to patients. Digitization has eased the works of healthcare professionals. The main motive of digital healthcare is to use the available resources to streamline the quality of medical assurance process, improve efficiency in digital healthcare and increase the accuracy of treatment [6].

1.3.4 Areas of Practice

Health informaticians perform research activities to investigate, find and improvise the process of health informatics. It involves providing solutions to various clinical, technical and organizational challenges that hamper the successful implementation of the system. According to American Medical Informatics Association (AMIA) [7], some of the practice areas that it supports are listed below:

1.3.4.1 Clinical Informatics

The use of information technology and informatics to provide healthcare services is termed as clinical informatics or operational informatics. It uses the domains of information technology, health system and clinical care and clinical informatics sits at the intersection of the above three domains. The primary focus is on healthcare data (i.e. individual patient's data) and use information technology as a medium to accomplish the goals. In clinical informatics, the specialist will work with clinical data from both clinical and healthcare informatics. It includes working with data entries and image storage systems on existing clinical practices.

1.3.4.2 Informatics in Clinical Research

Utilizing informatics to find and organize new knowledge related to disease and health is called clinical research informatics. It involves accumulating data obtained from clinical trials, translational activities, information management and informatics pertaining to use of clinical data in secondary research. It requires skill sets and predefined knowledge base that is not obtained in traditional school of medicine. Clinical informaticians improve patients care, community health outcomes and increase the clinician–patient relationship by analysing, designing, implementing and evaluating communication and information systems [8].

1.3.4.3 Informatics in Consumer Health

Informatics in consumer health is the subdomain of health informatics that aids in bridging the gap between patients and medical resources. The primary focus is on empowering the clients to manage their own health that include patient informatics,

Basics of Healthcare Informatics

health information literacy, consumer education and medical records and internet-based strategies. The new perspectives on informatics analyse the needs of consumers for information by studying and implementing methods that are accessible to consumers. Consumer informatics intersect with other fields such as nursing informatics, health promotion, public health education and communication science [7].

1.3.4.4 Informatics in Public Health

Public health informatics is another subdomain of health informatics that uses computer and information technology to support informatics in areas of public health. It includes learning, practice, surveillance, preparedness and research that applies to the promotion of public health.

1.3.4.5 Translational Bioinformatics (TB)

One of the youngest, emerging and interdisciplinary fields of health informatics that brings biological research into clinical informatics is called translational bioinformatics. It originates from biomedical data sciences that translates genetic, clinical and molecular data to treat the patient. The main goal is to use informatics methods to process the biomedical and genomic data to provide medical information and tools that physicians, researchers and patients can use. Bioinformatics knowledge bases use machine learning, data mining algorithms and other biostatistics techniques to build various prediction models improve human health care. Figure 1.2 [9] shows translational bioinformatics that bridges the gap between health informatics and bioinformatics.

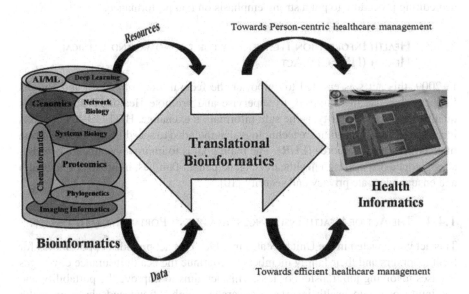

FIGURE 1.2 TB: A gap between Bioinformatics and Health Informatics [9].

1.4 LAWS IN HEALTH INFORMATICS

Due to rapid changes and technological evolution over the years, anyone who studies health informatics needs the most recent information to be ready to achieve the legal professional compliance because laws in health informatics are complex in nature. This section explores some major issues (ethics, patients' rights, responsibilities) of laws in health informatics that have been adopted in several countries.

1.4.1 THE 1974 PRIVACY ACT

The Privacy Act Law was enacted on 31 December 1974 by the U.S. Senate. This got commissioned to protect the individual privacy from exploitation through federal records. This law gives citizens the right to know what information is gathered about them to verify its accuracy and to request copies of data. These rules apply to the Indian health service and the veterans of health administration.

1.4.2 THE JOINT COMMISSION ACCREDITATION OF HEALTHCARE ORGANIZATIONS (JCAHO)

In 1951, a non-profit, private organization named the Joint Commission Accreditation of Healthcare Organizations (JCAHO) was established to assess and accredit facilities of hospitals and other healthcare organizations. The joint commission seeks to improve the public health care through evaluations and inspire health care organization to excel by providing effective care with highest quality values. In 1987, JCAHO introduced an agenda for change as an effort to develop a more advanced and modern accrediting procedure to put a strong emphasis on real performance.

1.4.3 HEALTH INFORMATION TECHNOLOGY FOR ECONOMIC AND CLINICAL HEALTH (HITECH) ACT

In 2009, this act was enacted to empower the federal wing of Health and Human Services that has the authority to supervise and promote Health IT that includes quality, safety and security as the safe information exchange. HITECH Act contains incentives related to healthcare technology that intended to speedup provider adoption of electronic health records (EHR). The main goal is to improve healthcare coordination, reduce disparities in healthcare, engage patient families, improve public health and ensure adequate privacy and security [10].

1.4.4 THE ACT OF HEALTH INSURANCE PRIVACY AND PORTABILITY (HIPPA)

This act was enacted in the United States in 1996. This act provides opportunities for health workers and their family members to continue the health insurance coverages in cases involving job transfers or loss. This act aims to improve the portability and continuity of group health insurance coverage, combat fraud and abuse in health insurance, improve access to long term services and coverage; and finally to improve the administration process of health insurance. Some standards were formed to enable

Basics of Healthcare Informatics

the identification of healthcare workers, health insurance firms and employers. One of the criteria is the National Provider Identifier Standard (NPIS), which assigns each medic a special number that is utilized in all facets of healthcare [11].

1.4.5 THE ACT OF PATIENT PROTECTION AND AFFORDABLE CARE (PPACA)

This act was enacted by the United States on 23 March 2010. This act was created with the intention of altering how people are insured and covered. The main objective is to bring down the healthcare costs so that coverage opens up to those who were previously uninsured. Major adjustments are being made to statue as problems with its application are discovered. The final decision should be anticipated as interpretation of its standards are created and implemented over the years [12].

1.4.6 THE ACT OF FOOD, DRUG ADMINISTRATION SAFETY AND INNOVATION (FDASIA)

The regulatory legislation of America was signed into law on 9 July 2012. The United States Food and Drug Administration (FDA) collects revenue from the medical industry, which reinforces the objective of the agency to protect public health by collecting fees from generic drug, medical devices and biological products. It creates a supervisory framework for health IT to augment mobile application and increase patient safety and innovation in the delivery of healthcare. The field of health informatics is affected by several state and federal regulations. Each law relates to patient care that gathers and maintains patient records. Understanding these laws and their ramification is key for better performance in the creation and promotion of computer-based patient care systems [13].

1.4.7 MEDIA CARE ACCESS AND CHIP REAUTHORIZATION ACT (MACRA)

This act came into existence in 2015 with the bipartisan support of U.S. legislature. It offered a new structure for the physicians, which demonstrates value over volume in the patient care. One of the primary provisions of this act is to upsurge fair funding to the clinicians and doctors. It strengthened the Medicare access through sustainable growth by improving physician's payments to reauthorize Children Health Insurance Programs (CHIP). The regulations related to MACRA also cover financial incentives for doctors and other providers to use health IT. Clinicians also took part in the excellence payment program using either advanced alternative payment model (APM) or Merit based Incentive Payment System (MIPS). Additionally, MACRA will integrate present quality reporting programs into single unified system [10, 14, 15].

1.5 CHALLENGES IN HEALTH INFORMATICS

The extended type of information science and information engineering branch gives rise to health informatics. Information processing and information systems engineering are addressed in this field. The integration of experiences, boundaries,

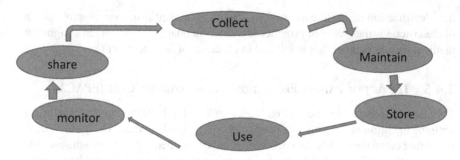

FIGURE 1.3 Health information lifecycle [5].

connections, controlled networks and emerging technologies are related to health information relation through this field. This led to the assessment of informatics with social, natural, statistical and computational perspective, including the study of social effect. So, the health informatics is a widespread area which contains information systems, statistics and data science.

The use of computer in the medical sector has a long history and in the present day, it is increasing more and more. Since health informatics is an advanced extension of health records in electronic form and health data analytics system, it is very helpful for utilizing the innovative technologies to improve the healthcare system. Research has been done to deliver a chronicle of evolution of the HL7 (Health Level 7) messaging standards, an introduction to HL7 FHIR (Fast Health Interoperability Resources) and a comparative analysis between HL7 FHIR and previous HL7 messaging standards [1]. The present-day healthcare system uses available information technology and deals with health records. It helps in creating, analysing and organizing health records. It helps in managing, storing, recovering and utilizing the data in health and medication. And the medical records will be available to patients, doctors, nurses, caregivers and also to the stakeholders whoever require the data. So health informatics can also be called as biomedical informatics. It should be stressed that health informatics is not a technology whereas it is related to health. The medical record has been collected, processed, used, analysed, shared and stored. Health informatics adds new opportunities, greater availability, lower cost, higher efficiency and quality to the existing healthcare system. It is also an emerging specialization for improving the safety and quality of patients, which combines information technology, communications and healthcare. It also includes a group of methodologies to manage information in the health sector and it improves the data management of patients [2, 4]. Figure 1.3 shows the lifecycle of health information.

There are several challenges faced during research in health informatics [5] and we will highlight a few important ones.

1.5.1 Conventional Healthcare Environment

It is a troublesome adventure to change to new models of reliable information because of the present timetables from production to execution. This is implied by existing administrative conditions. The trusted and reliable connections are the important aspects among all the devices to excel in health informatics. The limits in the present-day scenarios are due to expanding contactedness and the reduction of authoritative limits [6].

1.5.2 Design of Infrastructure

The infrastructure requirement for the health informatics is high due to the requirement of storing a large amount of data. So these expectations bring more security challenges and problems. The issue in the infrastructure is of dynamic or static network. The communication for moving the messages safely may not work properly. Therefore, there are critical difficulties in the security, assurance and administration of this information [7]. Presently the associations are mainly dependent on trust. There may be threats of cyber-attacks, which may not be considered by the medical device engineer [8].

1.5.3 Interoperability Issue

The data exchanging standards continue to evolve and due to the use of different wearable devices in health informatics. So providing interoperability among various types of devices is a big issue. The system should be interoperable in such a way that the data should be transferred among all the devices and also among multiple interfaces where the device needs to be compatible with one another. It is important to consider that the combination of interfaces used for communication between multiple systems is almost double. There is no information available regarding the capability of the devices in the network. Device conventions, functionality, standards and phrasing indexes are required in the device registry. So the device diversity, interoperability and vulnerability issues arise in the health informatics [16].

1.5.4 Consistency and Integrity of Data

Providing data integrity is a big problem in health informatics. Data integrity is the overall accuracy, consistency and completeness of data. That means preserving original data from alterations. If the system provides data integrity, then it guarantees the correctness of data by minimizing the errors and therefore it improves the safety of patients. Presently, the approved clients are also making mistakes due to their incomplete knowledge about the system. The system has become inconsistent because everybody is using different features of the system without complete knowledge about the system. One of the most important challenges for health informatics is that it has to deal with a huge amount of data [17]. Heterogeneous data due to different systems is one more biggest challenges we face in these systems [18].

1.5.5 Data Access Control

Data access is the on-demand availability to copy, modify, retrieve or move data from the health information system by an authorized user. The privacy and security of any data can be ensured by controlling the access to information. The control over the complete system is mandatory for health informatics. It can be provided by enabling different access segmentation to the complete system. It is very important to manage all the data complying with the rules and regulations of the government and also to protect vital information about the patients from unauthorized access. The patient provides the data. The responsibility of the system is to build up this data, which is essential for securing the system from unauthorized access and to protect the patient's health-related information from manipulation. Other than patients, the supervisors who are also the staff who takes care of the patients in the health organization can access data [19]. Access control is very much important for providing authorization. The health record stored in the cloud can be disseminated over large area and providing security for this data can be a big challenge for the system.

1.5.6 Human Factors

A huge role is played by human beings in using health Informatics. Because of this, the staff need to be trained before developing the technology. A usability study has to be conducted before developing and adopting a new system of human informatics. A research study was conducted by KTH University and it has proved the human challenge in 76% of the times [20]. The result also discusses several access control models and their merits and demerits and also the roles to encourage privacy in cloud-based solutions.

1.5.7 Privacy Concerns

The ultimate use of information by a substantial number of people in the area leads to the expansion of the data. A few number of datasets are openly accessible whereas different kinds of information have many degrees of confidentiality concerns. The health information is a very sensitive information and providing privacy to the data is very important aspect of this system. Only approved staff must be able to access it [21]. Privacy is a vital concern in the healthcare sector and it has to be provided correctly and wrong handling of privacy may also lead to death of the patient if the required information is not provided on time. The health of the patients must be monitored at regular intervals [22]. The privacy breaches are very important concerns and it will cause different types of damages [23].

1.5.8 Data Authenticity

Authenticity means the true validity of data. Authentic data is the accurate and truthful data. Authenticity is very much required in any communication. Without authentication, there may be chances of mam in the middle attack. Endpoint authentication is required to prevent this type of attack.

1.5.9 Laws and Ethics

Laws are the rules made to mandate or prohibit certain behaviours of the society. They are drawn from ethics. The ethics define socially acceptable behaviours. Laws carry the sanctions of a governing authority and ethics are based on the cultural facts. Sometimes laws and ethics lead to privacy violations. Hospitals and government provide data about the patients and their diseases to research organizations so that it will aid in case of a disease outbreak. Law and ethics have to ensure responsible use of data by research agencies and without misusing it.

1.5.10 Confidentiality and Availability

Confidential data is the one which is not readable by any other middle person. Authorization provides confidentiality to the data. Data will be made available only to the authorized person. Authorization to the data is provided depending on the role of the person in the organization. Thus, nothing will be shared without the consent of the patient. The system should be designed in such a way that whenever the doctor wants the data, it should be available.

1.6 EMERGING TECHNOLOGIES IN HEALTH INFORMATICS

Technological advancement has revolutionized healthcare by sparking innovation across all medical disciplines. The ongoing developments completely rely on various technologies that combine industry-wide innovations that transform the healthcare field. This section throws light on some of the emerging technologies which are widely used in health informatics.

1.6.1 Blockchain

The biggest challenge in health informatics is to integrate information technology in medical design to accurately deliver health care services at the right time. It involves acquisition, storage, processing, distribution and retrieval of healthcare data to collaborate between healthcare providers and patients [24].

Blockchain is one such emerging technology that provides a high level of transparency and security across medical informatics. It is a decentralized distributed network that protects the confidential medical data. Each blockchain network contains a chain of blocks that are controlled through a genesis block. All transactions of digital ledger can be verified through the genesis block (publicly registered and checked). The data registered through transaction requires a great deal of accountability. To modify or delete the medical data, each block in the Blockchain network reaches a consensus that prevents other blocks to tamper contents. Once medical data are written in the Blockchain, nobody can modify that data and it remains intact and unchanged. This way Blockchain secures and strengthens the system. The falsification causes of health informatics can be easily discovered through Blockchain. All medical history, diverse illness patients records, therapies and medication details can be easily stored on the Blockchain network without actually being modified, thus improving stability and less prone to hacker attacks [25].

For example, the United States National Library of Medicine adopted Blockchain technology to improve insurance claim process, manage medical records, accelerate biomedical and clinical research and manage healthcare data ledgers.

1.6.2 ARTIFICIAL INTELLIGENCE AND MACHINE LEARNING (AI AND ML)

One of the buzzwords in the computer science domain that gained attention in biomedicine healthcare, medical education and other industry is artificial intelligence (AI) and machine learning. The term AI mimics the real human intelligence. Artificial intelligence has numerous applications in diverse fields such as information technology, banking, education and healthcare. Modern AI and machine learning tools, models and technologies aid in the rapid detection, diagnosis and treatment of a vast range of diseases such as cancer, pneumonia, diabetes and neurodegenerative diseases. In order to help medical professionals attain diagnostic precision and anticipate probable high-risk illnesses, AI and ML are being used in the fields of healthcare and health informatics. Some of application areas of AI in medical domain are health monitoring, radiology, surgery, manage patient data, drug discovery, remote consultation, personalized treatments, medical statistics and imaging. Artificial intelligence and machine learning attract scientists, researchers to carry out research and innovations from diverse disciplines that includes computer science, social science, business, biology and medicine [26].

For example, AI-based platforms help to simplify, improve and optimize the work of a cardiologist. The biomedical data collected automatically from cardiac patients through mobile sensors helps the cardiologist to capture, analyse, monitor, interpret and visualize data to diagnose the problems of heart failure based on patient history, physical examinations and laboratory reports (case study of Attia et al., an application of AI to electrocardiogram (ECG) for measuring heart electrical activity).

1.6.3 CLOUD COMPUTING

The technological evolution and rapid growth of digital data has had a significant impact on healthcare services. In many developed countries, the usage of IT in the medical domain had led to a significant improvement in the health care provision services. Cloud computing is one method of delivering computing resources and services. Cloud computing is one such evolving technology that had brought benefits to the medical systems for integrating resources. Cloud computing enables to deploy remote servers through use of internet that can manage, store and process healthcare data. Cloud computing enables customers to make use of applications and network-based tools through a web browser, which creates the illusion that the programs and applications are installed on their own computer. To address the escalating challenges, health care providers find productive innovative and cost-effective methods. The use of cloud computing eases the work of clinicians, doctors, pharmacy and health insurance facilitators by granting access to comprehensive medical data (electronic health records) by alerting and reducing prescription errors [27, 28].

For example, The Aurum Institute used IBM Watson cloud computing and data analytics technologies to collect all clinical data to improve the efficiency and accuracy of the captured data. The optimization of data helped Aurum Institute to quickly determine actionable outcomes.

Basics of Healthcare Informatics

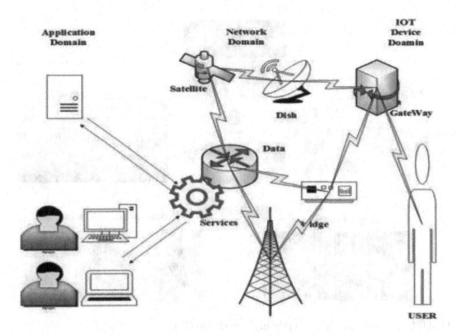

FIGURE 1.4 IOT Communication with other networking devices [29].

1.6.4 IOT AND INTERNET OF MEDICAL OF THINGS (IOMT)

Over the last few decades, we have witnessed tremendous surge in the research and development of instruments and devices that could operate using the internet. The Internet of Medical Things emerged as one such area that has changed the face of healthcare sector. In simpler terms, it is one such technology that connects medical devices and instruments to healthcare systems through internet. The use of WiFi helps to send the signals wirelessly to connect medical devices and instruments. Figure 1.4 [29] illustrates how IOT communicates with other network devices.

The Internet of Medical Things uses many healthcare apps that aid in monitoring the patient health by gathering medical data. It also records and maintains exact data on patients with fewer mistakes. All medical staff and doctors can now gather patient information and store it in the cloud through Internet of Medical Things [29].

For example, patients' health data can be sent to the doctors or health experts via Apple Watches, allowing the experts to examine real-time data and provide better solutions for the patients (i.e., real-time data care system) [30].

1.6.5 3D PRINTING

In the year 1980, the concept of 3D printing was first introduced. 3D printing can be formally defined as "The process of creating a 3D solid object of virtually any shape to form a digital model." Recently, 3D printing has gained significant attention from researchers in the field of biomedical applications. Around the world, many

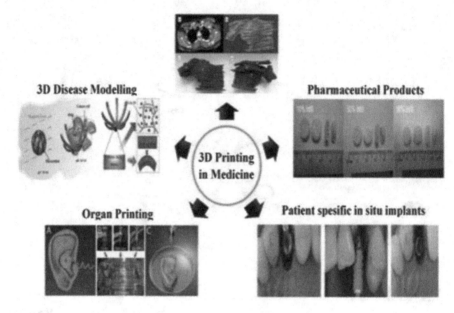

FIGURE 1.5 Application of 3D printing in medicine [31].

companies have invested in and significantly contributed to the use of manufacturing methods in medical domains through their laboratories and scientific research. The advancement of medical system and high-tech devices had the potential to create customized prosthetics, anatomical models, implants, tissue-organ fabrication and customized medical products. These are some of the major applications of 3D printing that have revolutionized industry. Figure 1.5 shows applications of 3D printing in medicine [31].

For example, a polish company introduced the first 3D printer called "Zortrax," which was evaluated by the users of 3Dhubs site [32, 33]. Using a 3D printed replica of donor kidney, Belfast surgeons successfully trained for a kidney transplant on a 22-year-old woman in January 2018 [34].

1.6.6 Nanomedicine

One of the new, fast-growing areas that has gained the attention of the research community over the years is the nanomedicine technology. Nanomedicine uses the science of nanotechnology that is applied to healthcare applications for the diagnosis and treatment of various diseases using nanoparticles, biosensors and molecular nanotechnology. Nanomedicine has brought new therapeutic approaches and diagnostic innovations to a variety of medical domains. Nanomedicine uses nanoparticles or molecules in drugs to improve tissue and specific cells that are produced at the nanoscale level and are safe to be introduced into the human body. In a broader sense of project, nanomedicine projects are comparable to other medical and industrial projects; yet due to their special characteristics, extra components are included in the

Basics of Healthcare Informatics

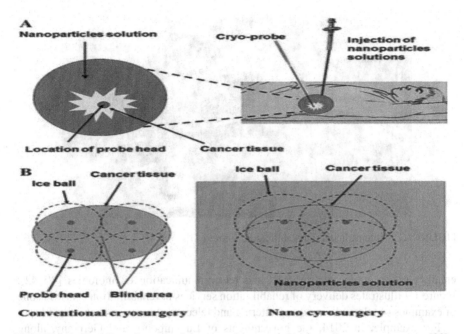

FIGURE 1.6 Loading of nanoparticles around cancer tissue through nano-cryosurgery [38].

project stream. A lot of avenues in nanomedicine research have attracted researchers who gained insight into nanomedicine projects that are categorised based on several factors. These categories include nano sensors, nano imagers, nano tissues, nano robots, nano instruments, nano drugs and nano fibres [35–38]. Figure 1.6 shows nano-cryosurgery that loads specific nanoparticles around the cancer tissue.

For example, the scientists of Nova Nordisk and MIT Engineers have designed and developed a smart pill called "PillCam – A capsule" that contains a miniature video camera that uses nanotechnology to perform advanced functions such as sensing, imaging and drug delivery [39].

1.6.7 Telemedicine

Over the last two centuries, telemedicine has made significant contributions and advancements in the field of healthcare domain. To overcome the global problems of quality and accessibility of healthcare services, proper implementation of telemedicine is required in healthcare. Telemedicine can be formally defined as any form of virtual communication that happens between doctors and patients through the use of communication and information technology. It allows the exchange of information from one site to another through the use of electronic media, which enables doctors, patients and medical professionals to interact through video conferencing, eliminating the need for physical interactions. Telemedicine is a boon to millions of people who live in remote locations and lack medical and transportation facilities. Telemedicine has multiple application with different services such as computers,

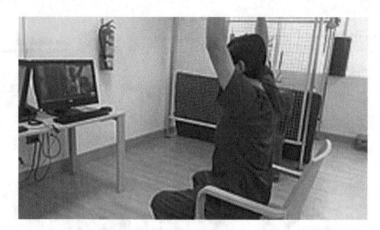

FIGURE 1.7 Telemedicine in rehabilitation centres [43].

email, wireless tools, smartphones and telecommunication technologies [40–42]. Figure 1.7 illustrates delivery of rehabilitation services in rehabilitation centres is one of examples of telemedicine using internet and telecommunications networks [43].

For example, in 2014, the governments of Luxembourg and Germany, along with few nongovernmental organizations, medical doctors and health professionals launched SATMED (Satellite based eHealth Communication Platform), a health app aimed at improving public health in remote areas of developing countries [44].

Telemedicine provides four major important benefits which includes

- Improving access care for the patients in the remote locations
- Improve cost effectiveness by reducing the cost of healthcare (short hospital stay, travel time reduction, professional healthcare staff sharing)
- Improve the quality of healthcare
- Increased support for telemedicine services and patient satisfaction (impacts on patients' family and community, less stress and travel time) [45].

1.6.8 BIG DATA ANALYTICS

One of the promising areas in the domain of computer science that has gained the attention of research community over the years is big data analytics. The widespread growth of communication and internet technologies has created voluminous amount of heterogeneous data. Many healthcare organizations proposed several models to support the best services and patient care. According to a survey conducted by International Data Corporation (IDC), the size of the data generated by digital universe is expected to grow to 40,000 Exa Bytes (EB) by the end of 2020 and continue to grow in the subsequent years. The properties of big data completely rely on major characteristics, which is also called 6V (velocity, volume, value, variability, veracity and variety). Based on the characteristics of big data, many open source processing platforms such as Hadoop, Hive, Cassandra and MapReduce provide support

Basics of Healthcare Informatics

to handle big data applications in medicine and healthcare sectors. Big data aims to collect, analyse and examine huge and varied data that helps organizations make business decisions by uncovering hidden patterns, finding unknown correlations and providing other useful information [46]. Data analytics helps the healthcare sector by analysing every aspect of patient care and operational management. These analyses help to investigate several methods to improve clinical care and enhance the efficiency of healthcare [47, 48].

1.6.9 Robotics

The evolution of the internet and advancements in AI technology have facilitated scientists and researchers who have transformed healthcare services through the use of intelligent robots. Because of the improved capabilities of artificial intelligence and machine learning, robotics equipped with AI capabilities that support administration, maintenance, surgical assistance, transportation and delivery play a significant role. To understand the behavioural needs of the users every day, AI provides support for better environment by offering guidance and through automated inputs. The capabilities of medical robots are being expanded through the use of AI and computer vision to support multiple areas of healthcare [49, 50].

1.7 APPLICATION OF HEALTH INFORMATICS

The growth of the medical domain, internet usage and developments in the communication network have had a significant impact on people's lives. The widespread use of various technologies has led to significant progress in healthcare and other application domains. This section throws some light on various applications of health informatics.

1.7.1 Ultrasound Imaging

The other name given for ultrasound imaging is sonography. Ultrasound imaging uses sound waves of high frequencies to capture the images of human organs in real time that shows movement of flow of blood inside the blood veins. Unlike X-ray imaging, with ultrasound imaging, there is no ionising radiation exposure. Ultrasound imaging is performed by inserting a transducer (probe) into a body opening or on top of the skin by injecting gel into the body. The ultrasound image is created based on the reflection of body waves structures. The information required to create an image is provided by the strength (amplitude) of the sound signal and the time it takes for the wave to travel through the body. Ultrasound imaging is considered to be much more secure than X-ray imaging because it is based on non-ionized radiation. Although it is considered safe, it tends to have some biological effects on the body. It can heat up the tissue cells and produce small pockets of gas in the body fluids or tissues or cavitation [51]. Figure 1.8a and 1.8b depict the use of a transducer probe during a routine ultrasound examination to monitor and assess foetus and mother health during pregnancy.

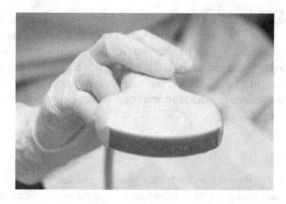

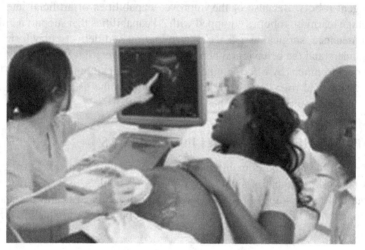

FIGURE 1.8 (a) and (b) Use of a transducer probe during a routine ultrasound examination to monitor and assess the foetus and mother's health during pregnancy [51].

1.7.2 CT Imaging

It is one of the medical imaging techniques that uses computerized X-ray imaging, in which a narrow beam of X-ray light is quickly rotated around the human body. This produces computer signals that are analysed by the computer to create cross-sectional images or slices of the patient's body. These slices are called tomographic images. The computer collects these successive slices that are stacked together to form a 3D image of the patient for easy identification of tumours or any other abnormalities. CT imaging of the head is done to locate the internal injuries, tumours, haemorrhage, blood clot cells, excess fluid and clots leading to strokes and also presence of tumours. CT imaging aids in the diagnosis of life-threatening disease conditions such as cancer, haemorrhage and severe blood clot that can save human lives. When exposed to ionizing radiations, CT imaging produces ionizing radiations, which can cause biological effects in the living human tissues. It can even cause allergic reactions

Basics of Healthcare Informatics

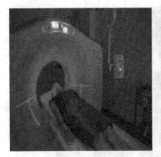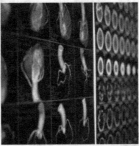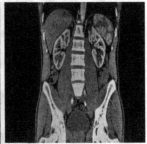

FIGURE 1.9 Images of patients inside CT machine and CT images of (a) heart, (b) coronary artery and (c) abdomen [52].

in some patients, and in rare cases, leads to temporary kidney failure. The researchers of the National Institute of Biomedical Imaging and Bioengineering (NBIB) [52] developed image reconstruction techniques to efficiently triage patients with stroke symptoms. Figure 1.9a shows images of patients inside CT machine and CT images of heart, coronary artery (Figure 1.9b) and abdomen (Figure 1.9c)

1.7.3 Magnetic Resonance Imaging (MRI)

It is one of the non-invasive medical imaging techniques used in radiology that produces three-dimensional detailed anatomical images which are used to diagnose the disease and guide treatment. It is a sophisticated technology that excites and detects changes in the direction of the rotational axis of protons that makes up a living tissue. MRI scanners use strong magnetic fields that uses the radio waves to generate the images of the organs in the body. MRI, unlike CT imaging, doesn't use ionizing radiation, which helps to improve the contrast of the images of soft tissues. The powerful magnets of MRI enable to provide a resilient magnetic field that forces protons to get aligned with that field at specific angles of 90 degrees or 180 degrees when a radiofrequency field is turned off. The MRI sensors will detect the energy released by the protons that gets realigned with the magnetic field. Although MRI doesn't emit ionizing radiation, the strong magnetic field created by these machines can exert forces on magnetisable objects, causing twitching sensations when nerves are stimulated. Figure 1.10a and 1.10b shows study images of head and abdomen of patient positioned for MRI [53, 54].

1.7.4 Diagnosis of Cancer

One of the promising application areas in the domain of medical informatics that has gained the attention of researchers is cancer diagnosis. In the treatment of cancer and research, storing, extracting and encoding information plays a key role. The healthcare data stored in electronic systems follows different formats: structured or unstructured. The prime goal is to organize the data that is comprehensive and significant to researchers, patients and clinicians. The advancement of communication and

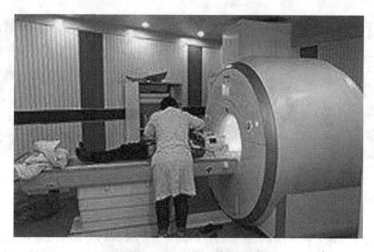

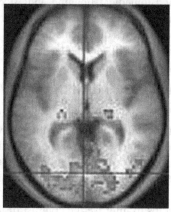

FIGURE 1.10 (a) and (b) Study images of head of patient position for MRI [53, 54].

information technologies has brought major benefits to cancer diagnosis research. From the health informatics perspective, several tools and techniques enhance the categorisation and accessibility of oncological data, improving the effectiveness of cancer diagnosis and treatments. Based on the pre-existing features collected from medical images, majority of AI supported imaging applications concentrate on early screening and diagnosis. Figure 1.11 depicts the complete summary of cancer informatics using Artificial Intelligence [55].

1.7.5 Development of Drugs

Over the past few years, the drug discovery process and computer technologies have co-evolved, making them inseparable components and creating a pipeline for basic research ending with the creation of pharmaceuticals. The development and discovery of drug is a complex process that generates enormous volumes of

Basics of Healthcare Informatics

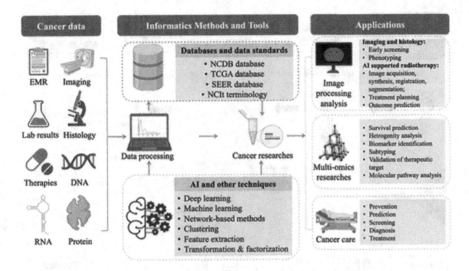

FIGURE 1.11 Summary of cancer informatics using Artificial Intelligence [55].

data and information. The core components of drug discovery process involve the use of computer technologies for the prediction of the drug's chemical structure, pattern discovery, molecular modelling and access of heterogeneous database. The use of drug discovery informatics minimizes the amount of time required for researching a drug that hit the market. There are seven stages in the drug discovery process:

- Selection of the disease
- Target hypothesis
- Lead compound identification
- Lead optimization
- Preclinical trial testing
- Clinical trial testing
- Pharmacogenomics optimization and post marketing

Each of the above steps involves complex scientific interactions that uses information technology components that helps execution [56–58].

Figure 1.12a and 1.12b shows various stages of drug discovery process along with preclinical research studies [56–58].

1.8 RESEARCH AVENUES IN HEALTH INFORMATICS

Health informatics is a diverse field that has expanded over the years, attracting the research community. Increased patients' data and technological advancements in health informatics will improve the state of the healthcare system. This section lists some of the research areas in health informatics [59–61].

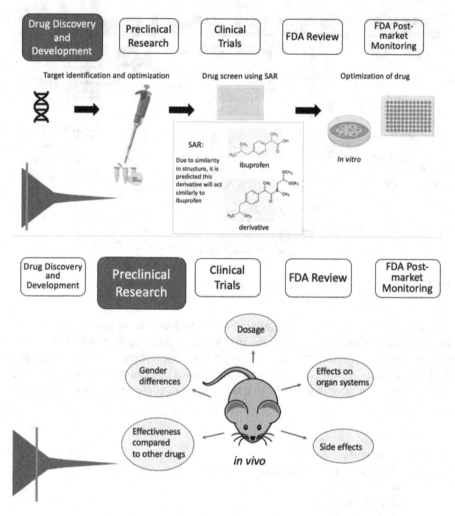

FIGURE 1.12 (a) Stages of discovery of drug process [54–56], (b) Preclinical research studies of drug discovery [56–58].

- Electronic health Records (EHR)
- Biomedical ontologies and standards
- Consumer health informatics
- Telemedicine
- Mobile health
- Clinical decision support systems and clinical tools
- Intelligent systems
- Informatics in health care modelling
- Precision medicine
- Wearable technologies

Basics of Healthcare Informatics

- Augmented reality, virtual reality and mixed reality
- Education and training in cross reality
- Data analytics
- Natural language processing and text and data mining

1.9 CASE STUDIES

Case studies are the best ways to better understand any system that enables detailed examination of a particular case in a real-world context. This section sheds light on two important cases in field of healthcare.

1.9.1 Use of Augment Reality to Make Learning Easier in Oral Histology

Histology or microscopic anatomy is branch of biology that studies the microscopic anatomy of biological tissues using a microscope. Any person who studies tissues, genetic, cells and organs for diagnosis is termed as histopathologist. This is widely adopted in the field of medicine, dental and healthcare sciences. Classroom instructions are supplemented with a microscopic laboratory component in a traditional instruction. To comprehend the microanatomy, development of tooth and oral structures, the University of Alberta students majoring in dentistry and dental hygiene spend a lot of time studying oral histology. The School of Dentistry uses PowerPoint presentations with photos of textbooks to teach oral histology with the help of light microscopy labs. The main expectation of students is to recognize the histological section by identifying the structural components. A special application utilizing the augment reality is required to facilitate learning outside of class time with practice labelled photomicrographs. Figure 1.13 shows images of AR phone application Dental AR that helped students to learn and understand model of cellular structure at their own pace.

The Dental AR uses the information and communication technology that has a digital database consists of heterogeneous oral histology images that includes different tooth structures, tooth palates, oral mucosa, salivary glands, cell layers and other types of oral structures. Unity 3D was used to develop Dental AR with Vuforia.

During the corona pandemic, the oral histology training was provided to first-year dentistry students in an online mode. Virtual meetings encouraged the students to download and use the dental augmented reality application. The board images are posted on the online learning management system with a set of practice questionnaire that enabled students to use Dental AR for practising oral histology using their cell phone at their own pace. Figure 1.14 shows the photomicrographs of target images of Dental AR application that depicts teeth, oral structures, tooth and facial developments, oral mucosa and salivary glands.

The major drawback is that not all students will have the privilege to access these type of technologies. Another drawback of using this technology for learning is the distraction of using a smartphone. Despite these pitfalls, Dental AR provided promising future to facilitate effective learning [62].

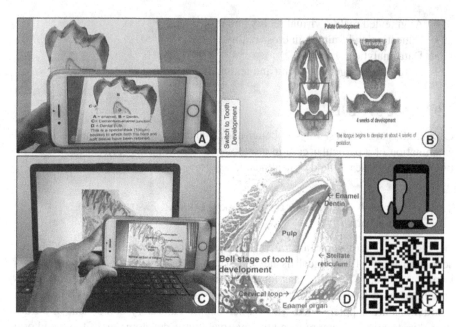

FIGURE 1.13 Dental AR Phone application to understand cellular structure [62].

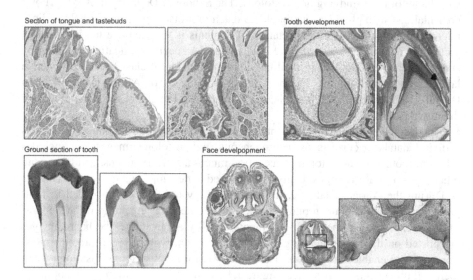

FIGURE 1.14 Photomicrographs of tooth and other structures in Dental AR application [62].

1.9.2 Aortic Valve Surgery Using Three-Eyed Endoscope

The primary predisposing factors for heart disease such as smoking, high cholesterol and high blood pressure, have all increased significantly in the population over the subsequent years. In the western world, aortic stenosis (AS) is considered as the third most common type of heart disease with a 50% chance of mortality within three years on the production of symptoms. AS develops as a result of leaflets gradual calcification, which over time reduces the aperture to the point where the valve is no longer able to regulate the flow of blood. This usually appears above the age of 65 at a high percentage of 21–26.

The only treatment is to have aortic valve replacement (AVR). For severe AS, the surgical AVR has been considered as the standard treatment. The open heart technique in traditional surgery gives surgeon a blunt access to the heart through median sternotomy. But despite access to cardiac structures, heart requires a complete dissection of sternum, thus disrupting the wall of chest. Many robotic systems assisted the cardiac surgery. This study aims to implement the AVR using three-eyed endoscope [63].

Figure 1.15 illustrates the usage of platform to conduct aortic valve surgery using three-eyed endoscope technology. The surgeon uses a pair of joysticks that act as a control unit to operate the robots that is held by the place holder. In the proposed surgical scenario, flexible manipulator is attached to the actuator that is fixed by the holder that gets attached to the patient's bed. This flexible manipulator has omni bending capabilities, which are connected and controlled by four sets of cables and servo motors. The holder gets connected by three endoscopic cameras. Surgeons

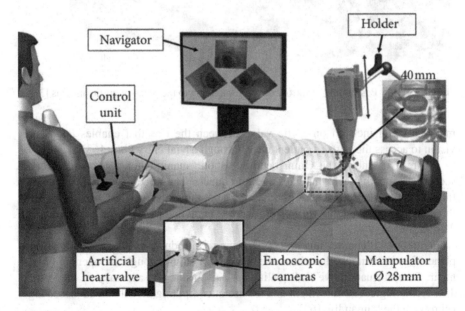

FIGURE 1.15 Aortic valve surgery using three eye endoscope [63].

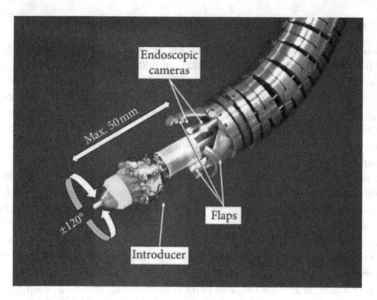

FIGURE 1.16 Robotic manipulator consisting of endoscopic cameras [3].

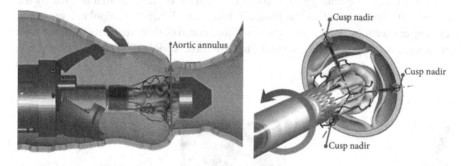

FIGURE 1.17 Positioning of introducer corresponding to the plane of aortic annulus [3].

makes a small incision on aortic valve between the ribs that enables endoscopic vision to access the parts of patient chest through trivial entry point [63].

Figure 1.16 shows the Omni bending robotic manipulator consisting of endoscopic cameras that contains flaps and introducers. The three flaps are opened when the manipulator is too close to the heart. The complete surgery is carried out using three endoscopic cameras with a 120-degree manipulator having a circumference of 21 mm [63].

Figure 1.17 illustrates how the positioning of introducer sits corresponding to the plane of aortic annulus that clears the cholesterol clogs through the opening of cusp nadir. Several quantitative and qualitative tests ensure the accuracy of the system. This technological advancement and the use of computing model and advanced algorithm save the human life [63].

1.10 CONCLUSION

Health informatics is one of the emerging technologies in the field of medicine that has caught the attention of many technologists, developers and researchers over the years. The rapid advancements in the domains of health informatics have created new ways of assessment methods for the interpretation of patient data with the use of scientific research. Health informatics is not restricted only to applications, computer or information management in healthcare. The prime focus of this chapter aimed at providing a comprehensive overview about the health informatics that emphasize practice area of health informatics across several sectors. It also highlights various laws of health informatics by highlighting the challenges. It also talked about various emerging technologies in health informatics in diverse fields of healthcare. Lastly it touched on some of applications of informatics in various sectors. Finally, the research avenues of health informatics along with some case studies are discussed in detail.

REFERENCES

[1] Michael Imhoff. "Health informatics." *Evaluating Critical Care* (2002): 255–269.

[2] Bryant and Stratton College Blog Staff. URL: www.bryantstratton.edu/blog/2017/october/what-are-health-informatics

[3] Cynthia S. Gadd, Elaine B. Steen et al. "Domains, tasks, and knowledge for health informatics practice: results of a practice analysis." *Journal of the American Medical Informatics Association* 27(6) (June 2020): 845–852, https://doi.org/10.1093/jamia/ocaa018

[4] Branko Cesnik, E. Hovenga, M. Kidd, Churchill Livingstone. "Health informatics: An overview." eHealth Ebook, URL: www.achi.org.au/docs/HNI_Book/

[5] Donghua Chen and Runtong Zhang. "Exploring research trends of emerging technologies in health metaverse: A bibliometric analysis" (5 January 2022). Available at SSRN: https://ssrn.com/abstract=3998068 or http://dx.doi.org/10.2139/ssrn.3998068

[6] R.L. Richesson, J.E. Andrews, et al. "Introduction to clinical research informatics." In: R. Richesson and J. Andrews, (eds), *Clinical Research Informatics. Health Informatics*. Springer, Cham (2019). https://doi.org/10.1007/978-3-319-98779-8_1

[7] "Informatics: Research and practice." 2022. AMIA – American Medical Informatics Association. https://amia.org/about-amia/why-informatics/informatics-research-and-practice

[8] Duane Bender, Sartipi et al. HL7 FHIR: An agile and RESTful approach to healthcare information exchange. Proceedings of CBMS 2013 – 26th IEEE International Symposium on Computer-Based Medical Systems, pp. 326–331 (2013). 10.1109/CBMS.2013.6627810

[9] Edward H. Shortliffe et al. *Computer Applications in Health Care and Biomedicine*. Springer, Heidelberg (2006).

[10] M.F. Collen. "The origins of informatics." *Journal of American Medical Informatics Association* 1(2) (1994): 91–107.

[11] E. Coiera, E. Ammenwerth, Georgiou et al. "Does health informatics have a replication crisis?" *Journal of American Medical Informatics Association* 25(8) (2018): 963–968.

[12] J. Nguyen, L. Smith et al. "Conventional and complementary medicine health care practitioners' perspectives on interprofessional communication: A qualitative rapid review." *Medicina (Kaunas)* 55(10) (2019): 650. doi: 10.3390/medicina55100650. PMID: 31569742; PMCID: PMC6843134.

[13] P.A.H. Williams, McCauley et al. "Always connected: the security challenges of the healthcare Internet of Things." In: 2016 IEEE 3rd World Forum on Internet of Things (WF-IoT), Reston, VA, USA, pp. 30–35. https://doi.org/10.1109/wf-iot.2016.7845455 (2016)

[14] S.T. Argaw, J.R. Troncoso-Pastoriza, et al. "Cybersecurity of hospitals: Discussing the challenges and working towards mitigating the risks." *BMC Medical Informatics Decision Making* 20 (2020): 146. https://doi.org/10.1186/s12911-020-01161-7

[15] Shalini Bhartiya, Deepti Mehrotra, et al. "Challenges and recommendations to healthcare data exchange in an interoperable environment." *Electronic Journal of Health Informatics* 8 (2014) 1–24.

[16] "Important laws and regulations in health informatics." 2017. www.usfhealthonline.com/resources/health-informatics/important-laws-and-regulations-in-health-informatics/

[17] "Health insurance portability and accountability act – Wikipedia." 2010. https://en.wikipedia.org/wiki/Health_Insurance_Portability_and_Accountability_Act#HIPAA_acronym

[18] "Food and Drug Administration Safety and Innovation Act (FDASIA)." 2018. www.fda.gov/regulatory-information/selected-amendments-fdc-act/food-and-drug-administration-safety-and-innovation-act-fdasia

[19] Sara Rosenbaum, "The patient protection and affordable care act: Implications for public health policy and practice." *Public Health Reports* (Washington, D.C.: 1974) 126 (1) (2011): 130–135. doi: 10.1177/003335491112600118

[20] "Medicare Access and CHIP Reauthorization Act of 2015 – Wikipedia." 2017. https://en.wikipedia.org/wiki/Medicare_Access_and_CHIP_Reauthorization_Act_of_2015

[21] "What Is MACRA (Medicare Access and CHIP Reauthorization Act of 2015)? – Definition from WhatIs.Com." 2017. Search Health IT. www.techtarget.com/searchhealthit/definition/MACRA-Medicare-Access-and-CHIP-Reauthorization-Act-of-2015

[22] Abid Haleem, Mohd. Javaid, Ravi Pratap Singh, Rajiv Suman, and Shanay Rab. "Blockchain technology applications in healthcare: An overview." *International Journal of Intelligent Networks*, 2 (2021): 130–139. https://doi.org/10.1016/j.ijin.2021.09.005

[23] Bipin Kumar Rai. "Security issues and solutions for healthcare informatics." In *Federated Learning for IoT Applications*. Springer, Cham, pp. 185–198 (2022). doi:10.1007/978-3-030-85559-8_12

[24] Jonathan Mack. "10 Technologies that are changing health care." University of San Diego Online Degrees. 2016. https://onlinedegrees.sandiego.edu/8-technologies-changing-healthcare/

[25] "The importance of cloud computing in the healthcare industry." 2022. 3 December. https://neetable.com/blog/healthcare-industry-reliance-on-cloud-computing

[26] K. Jasim Omer, Safia Abbas, M. El-Sayed El-Horbaty, and M. Salem Abdel-Badeeh 2014. "Advent of cloud computing technologies in health informatics." Cloud Health Informatics, 9th International Conference, 21 November, pp. 31–39. www.researchgate.net/publication/267979291_ADVENT_OF_CLOUD_COMPUTING_TECHNOLOGIES_IN_HEALTH_INFORMATICS

[27] "Healthcare – products and platform." 2022. Apple (India). Accessed 3 December. www.apple.com/in/healthcare/products-platform/

[28] Gulraiz J. Joyia, M. Rao, Aftab Farooq Liaqat, and Saad Rehman. "Internet of Medical Things (IOMT): Applications, benefits and future challenges in healthcare domain." *Journal of Communications* 12(4) (2017): 240–247. doi:10.12720/jcm.12.4.240-247

[29] Helena Dodziuk. "Applications of 3D printing in healthcare." *Polish Journal of Thoracic and Cardiovascular Surgery* 13(2) (2016): 283–293. doi:https://doi.org/10.5114%2Fkitp.2016.62625
[30] "Zortrax Endureal." 2022. Zortrax. Accessed 3 December. https://zortrax.com/3d-printers/endureal/
[31] Allie Nawrat. 2018. "3D printing in the medical field: Four major applications revolutionising the industry." Medical Device Network. www.medicaldevice-network.com/features/3d-printing-in-the-medical-field-applications/
[32] Yahya Bozkurt and Elif Karayel. "3D Printing technology; Methods, biomedical applications, future opportunities and trends." *Journal of Materials Research and Technology* 14 (2021): 1430–1450. https://doi.org/10.1016/j.jmrt.2021.07.050
[33] "Nanotechnology in healthcare: 4 ways its changing the future." 2020. Netscribes. www.netscribes.com/nanotechnology-in-healthcare/
[34] Wilson Nwankwo, Akinola Samson Olayinka, and Kingsley E. Ukhurebor. "Nanoinformatics: Why design of projects on nanomedicine development and clinical applications may fail?" 2020 International Conference in Mathematics, Computer Engineering and Computer Science (ICMCECS), 1–8 May (2020). doi:10.1109/ICMCECS47690.2020.246992
[35] Wilson Nwankwo and Kingsley Eghonghon Ukhurebor. "Nanoinformatics: Opportunities and challenges in the development and delivery of healthcare products in developing countries." IOP Conference Series, *Earth and Environmental Science*, 655(1) (2020): 1–9. doi:10.1088/1755-1315/655/1/012018
[36] Vasanthi Vara. "Nanotechnology in medicine: Technology trends." Medical Device Network. (2020). www.medicaldevice-network.com/comment/nanotechnology-medicine-technology/
[37] Y. Wong, and Liu. 2012. "Nanomedicine: A primer for surgeons." *Pediatric Surgery International* 28(1): 943–951. doi: https://doi.org/10.1007/s00383-012-3162-y
[38] "Telehealth – Wikipedia." 2020. https://en.wikipedia.org/wiki/Telehealth
[39] "Telemedicine definition: What does telemedicine mean?" 2022. eVisit. Accessed 5 December. https://evisit.com/resources/telemedicine-definition
[40] "Satmed – Wikipedia." (2022). https://en.wikipedia.org/wiki/Satmed
[41] Andrea Moglia, Konstantinos Georgiou, Blagoi Marinov, Evangelos Georgiou, Raffaella Nice Berchiolli, Richard M SatavaMD, and Alfred Cuschier. "5G in healthcare: From COVID-19 to future challenges." *IEEE Journal of Biomedical and Health Informatics* 26(8) (2022): 4187–4196. doi:10.1109/JBHI.2022.3181205
[42] Dee Ford, Jillian B. Harvey, James McElligott, Kathryn King, Kit N. Simpson, Shawn Valenta, Emily H Warr, et al. "Leveraging health system telehealth and informatics infrastructure to create a continuum of services for COVID-19 screening, testing, and treatment." *Journal of the American Medical Informatics Association* 27(12) (2020): 1871–1877. https://doi.org/10.1093/jamia/ocaa157
[43] Zakir Haider, Bashaar Aweid, Padmanabhan Subramanian, and Farhad Iranpour. "Telemedicine in orthopaedics during COVID-19 and beyond: A systematic review." *Journal of Telemedicine and Telecare* 28(6) (2020): 391–403. doi:10.1177/1357633x20938241
[44] Blagoj Ristevski and Ming Chen. "Big Data analytics in medicine and healthcare." *Journal of Integrative Bioinformatics*, 15(3) (2018): 1–5. doi:10.1515/jib-2017-0030
[45] A.H. Gandomi, F. Chen, and L. Abualigah. "Machine learning technologies for big data analytics." *Electronics [Internet]* 11(3) (2022): 421. https://doi.org/10.3390/electronics11030421

[46] Sabyasachi Dash, Sushil Kumar Shakyawar, Mohit Sharma, and Sandeep Kaushik. "Big Data in healthcare: management, analysis and future prospects." *Journal of Big Data* 54(6) (2019): 1–25. doi:10.1186/s40537-019-0217-0

[47] Bikash Pradhan, Deepti Bharti, et al. "Internet of things and robotics in transforming current-day healthcare services." *Journal of HealthCare Engineering*, 15 (Special Issue) (2021): 1–15. Article ID 9999504. doi: https://doi.org/10.1155/2021/9999504

[48] Ashesh Shah. "AI & robotics in healthcare: Taking healthcare solutions to next dimension." Enterprise Mobility, Artificial Intelligence, Cloud, IoT, Blockchain Solutions & Services | Fusion Informatics Limited. 2020. www.fusioninformatics.com/blog/ai-robotics-in-healthcare-taking-healthcare-solutions-to-next-dimension/

[49] "Ultrasound imaging | FDA." 2020. www.fda.gov/radiation-emitting-products/medical-imaging/ultrasound-imaging

[50] "Computed Tomography (CT)." 2022. National Institute of Biomedical Imaging and Bioengineering. www.nibib.nih.gov/science-education/science-topics/computed-tomography-ct

[51] "Magnetic Resonance Imaging – Wikipedia." 2022. https://en.wikipedia.org/wiki/Magnetic_resonance_imaging

[52] "Magnetic Resonance Imaging (MRI)." 2022. National Institute of Biomedical Imaging and Bioengineering. Accessed 10 December. www.nibib.nih.gov/science-education/science-topics/magnetic-resonance-imaging-mri

[53] Na Hong, Gang Sun, Xiuran Zuo, Meng Chen, Li Liu, Jiani Wang, Xiaobin Feng, Wenzhao Shi, Mengchun Gong, and Pengcheng Ma. "Application of informatics in cancer research and clinical practice: Opportunities and challenges." *Cancer Innovation* 1(1) (2022): 80–91. doi:10.1002/cai2.9

[54] Devottam Gaurav, Fernando Ortiz Rodriguez, Sanju Tiwari, and M.A. Jabbar. *Review of Machine Learning Approach for Drug Development Process*, CRC Publishers, Boca Raton, FL, pp. 1–27 (2021). doi:10.1201/9781003161233-3

[55] Jeffrey Augen. "The Evolving role of information technology in the drug discovery process." *Drug Discovery Today* 7(5) (2002): 315–323. doi:10.1016/s1359-6446(02)02173-6

[56] (Amber) Ya LinChen. "Medical Informatics in Drug Discovery and Development." *Medium* (2021). https://bionewsdigest.medium.com/medical-informatics-in-drug-discovery-and-development-8849143e256a

[57] Kim Yong-Mi and Dursun Delen. "Medical informatics research trend analysis: A text mining approach." *Health Informatics Journal* 24 (4) (2016): 432–452. doi:10.1177/1460458216678443

[58] "What is health informatics? | Michigan Technological University." 2022. Michigan Technological University. Accessed 11 December. www.mtu.edu/health-informatics/what-is/

[59] "Health Informatics Research." 2022. Department of Health Administration and Policy. Accessed 11 December. https://hap.gmu.edu/academics/health-informatics/health-informatics-research

[60] Nazlee Sharmin, Ava K. Chow, Dominic Votta, and Nathanial Maeda. "Implementing augmented reality to facilitate the learning of oral histology." *Healthcare Informatics Research* 28(2) (2022): 170–175 (The Korean Society of Medical Informatics). doi:10.4258/hir.2022.28.2.170

[61] Virginia Mamone, Sara Condino, et al. "Low-computational cost stitching method in a three-eyed endoscope." *Journal of Healthcare Engineering*, (Special Issue) (2019): 1–12. Article ID 5613931. doi: https://doi.org/10.1155/2019/5613931

[62] Annette L. Valenta et al. "AMIA Board White Paper: AMIA 2017 core competencies for applied health informatics education at the master's degree level" *Journal of the American Medical Informatics Association*, 25(12) (2021): 1657–1668. www.researchgate.net/journal/Journal-of-the-American-Medical-Informatics-Association-1527-974X DOI: 10.1093/jamia/ocy132

[63] Sahar Qazi and Khalid Raza. "Translational bioinformatics in healthcare: Past, present, and future" *Translational Bioinformatics in Healthcare and Medicine*, 13 (2021): 1–12. https://doi.org/10.1016/B978-0-323-89824-9.00001-X

2 Foundation of Medical Data Sciences

S. M. Bramesh

2.1 INTRODUCTION

The Greek word *diabetes*, which means "to pass through," and the Latin word *mellitus*, which means "sweet," combines to form the name diabetes mellitus. A review of history suggests that Apollonius of Memphis coined the term "diabetes" sometime between 250 and 300 BC. The sweet character of urine in this illness was made aware of by ancient civilizations in India, Greece, and Egypt, and as a result, the term "diabetes mellitus" was popularized. Mering and Minkowski published on the role of the pancreas in the development of diabetes in 1889. The hormone insulin was isolated from a cow's pancreas by Collip, Banting, and Best at Toronto University in 1922, laying the path for a fruitful diabetic cure that same year. Excellent research has been done over the years, leading to several findings and the advancement of management methods to deal with this growing issue.

Diabetes is regrettably still one of the most common long-lasting diseases in the country and the world today [1, 2]. Globally, 415 million people (8.8% of the global population) have diabetes, and the International Diabetes Federation predicts that by 2020, that figure will rise to 642 million by 2030 [3]. Additionally, according to the World Health Organization (WHO), diabetes was the ninth major cause of death in 2019, accounting for roughly 1.5 million of the disease's direct fatalities.

Type 1 Diabetes (T1D), Type 2 Diabetes (T2D), young people with maturity-onset diabetes, pregnancy diabetes, neonatal diabetes, and alternate causes brought on by steroid usage, endocrinopathies, etc. are some of the several types of diabetes. The two main kinds of diabetes are T1D and T2D, which are primarily brought on by improper insulin release (T1D) and/or action (T2D). T2D is thought to affect older and middle-aged people with long-term hyperglycaemia as a result of poor nutritional and lifestyle decisions, whereas T1D is thought to affect adolescents or youngsters. However, all forms of diabetes carry a higher risk of overall premature death and can cause issues in numerous bodily regions. Possible outcomes include kidney failure, nerve damage, eyesight loss, leg amputation, and stroke. Furthermore, uncontrolled diabetes increases the risk of foetal death and other issues during pregnancy.

In comparison to people without diabetes, those with diabetes have a greater risk of developing a number of disorders [4]. Comorbidity is the term used in clinical literature to describe this phenomenon in general. Comorbidities make healthcare outcomes associated to diabetes, care requirements, treatment alternatives, and associated costs more difficult. Therefore, a thorough knowledge of the epidemiology of diseases co-occurring with diabetes is important for establishing treatment objectives.

The remaining sections of this chapter are as follows:

Section 2.2 reviews the applicability of EHRs in mining comorbidity patterns in diabetic patients and Section 2.3 briefly explains some of the challenges faced by the researchers to use EHR data. Section 2.4 provides details about different datasets and techniques used in the literature for mining comorbidity patterns in diabetic patients and Section 2.5 wraps up our discussion.

2.2 APPLICABILITY OF EHRS IN MINING COMORBIDITY PATTERNS IN DIABETIC PATIENTS

A longitudinal collection of electronic health data on specific patients and populations is referred to as an electronic health record [5]. Electronic health records are more comprehensive than paper records when it comes to patient data and medical treatment. EHRs are primarily used to record the healthcare process (for example, clinical care and billing).

The majority of contemporary electronic health record systems combine data from several sources, including pharmacy, nursing, administrative, radiology, laboratory, and physician entries, among others. Any department has the ability to produce electronic records. Hospitals and clinics may use a variety of supplementary systems from various vendors; in this scenario, the ancillary systems may or may not be integrated with the primary electronic health record system. These systems might be independent, and various vocabulary may have been employed. Data from these systems can be combined if the right interfaces are given; otherwise, to access the complete patient information, a doctor must open and log into several applications. Additionally, the total number of components in EHR could vary based on the service provided. Figure 2.1 displays several EHR system components.

For documenting the patient' state of health over time different types of data, including pictures, free-text, symbols, and numbers, can be stored in EHR systems. In summary, EHR contains mainly two types of data, namely unstructured and structured data. Demographics of patient (gender, age), weight, height, lab results, medications, and blood pressure are a few examples of structured data. Structured data types can be straightforwardly analysed using machine learning or conventional statistical techniques because the data already has a predetermined structure. However, due to the rapid growth of information on the patient's state, specialized knowledge for information extraction and analysis would be needed.

Contrarily, narrative data in EHRs, such as clinical notes, discharge summaries, surgical records, medical photographs, radiology reports, and pathology reports, is known as unstructured data [6]. Unstructured data can be used to extract a lot of valuable information, but doing so is more difficult because the data are not organized in a structured way. For instance, unstructured data, such as free-text summaries of

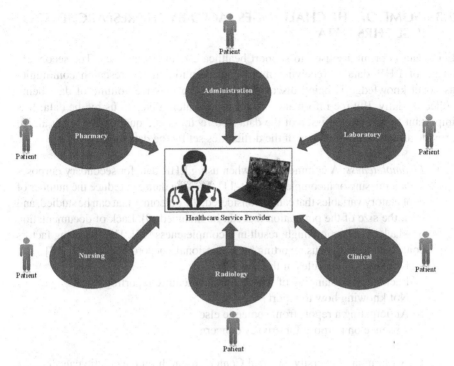

FIGURE 2.1 Electronic health record components.

discharge, comprise crucial details regarding the hospital stay or care episode, but it is challenging to extract this information since it is linked to several contexts and has a high degree of ambiguity. Furthermore, clinical texts include difficulties like ambiguities, spelling and grammatical errors, and abbreviations.

In conclusion, an EHR can have various presentations, data structures, and levels of detail based on the aim, service, location, and user's role. Ref. [7] is an example for the publicly accessible EHR system.

EHRs are beneficial for a variety of additional applications since they contain a wealth of relevant information. Examples include reducing medication errors, using efficient ways for clinician communication and information exchange, lowering healthcare expenses, improving the patients' medical records management, raising the standard of care, resulting in improved treatment [8], and enhancing population health in general. Last but not least, they may be modified to meet the needs of medical practice and are very adjustable.

The use of patient data that is regularly collected and kept to support research and create an epidemiological picture of disease is made possible by EHRs, which present an unmatched opportunity. Diabetes, in specific, stands to benefit, being a data-rich, chronic-disease state enabling researchers to conduct groundbreaking research in this domain.

2.3 SOME OF THE CHALLENGES FACED BY THE RESEARCHERS TO USE EHRS DATA

EHR data is primarily used to support healthcare-related functions. The secondary usage of EHR data is receiving more consideration in the research community as novel knowledge is being discovered due to the massive volume of data being collected daily. But the information is not immediately given to us by the data. It is important to address the issue of the data's correctness and quality. Beyley et al. [9] provide an outstanding review of the difficulties set by the data quality.

- *Incompleteness*: A common issue when using EHR data for secondary purposes is data missing or incompleteness [9–11]. Missing data can reduce the number of explanatory variables that can be considered, the outcomes that can be studied, and even the size of the population that can be included [9]. Lack of documentation or a lack of collection might result in incompleteness [12]. The following factors contribute to erroneous reporting by professionals, according to Hersh [13].
  - Oblivious to the rules of the law
  - Lack of understanding of which ailments require reporting
  - Not knowing how to report
  - Anticipating a report from someone else
  - Absence on purpose for privacy concerns

At the Columbia University Medical Center, research on pancreatic cancers utilizing International Classification of Diseases, Ninth Revision, Clinical Modification (ICD-9-CM) codes revealed that 48% of the patients' pathology reports lacked the associated diagnoses or disease evidence [14].

Incompleteness can also result from patients' inconsistent communication with the healthcare system. Certain tactics can be used to decrease the amount of missing data depending on the application, the type of data, and the percentage of missing data [12].

- *Erroneous data*: EHR data can also be inaccurate. Data are gathered from a variety of service areas, environmental factors, and geographical locations. Busy practitioners and staff gather EHR data. As a result, human error may have caused the data to be inaccurate. Erroneous data might also be produced by faulty equipment. Erroneous data should be located and corrected using validation techniques. Measures for external and internal validation can both be used. Internal validation can be used to determine whether data, such as inflated body mass index (BMI) or blood pressure readings, is credible. Dates can be used to determine whether a test actually occurred before the result that was generated. Data comparison with other patients or historical values is a form of external validation.
- *Uninterpretable data*: It's possible that some of the acquired EHR data won't be understandable. It has a close relationship to data incompletion. It could happen when only a portion of the data is collected and the remainder is not. For instance, it will be challenging to evaluate the result value if no specified quantitative or qualitative measuring unit is provided.

Foundation of Medical Data Sciences 39

- *Inconsistency*: Data inconsistency has a significant impact on analysis and outcome. Inconsistency may result from changes in data gathering methods, coding conventions, and standards over time and between different institutions. This problem may frequently arise in multi-institutional studies, particularly because many healthcare facilities use various suppliers to supply equipment, software, and other technology [9]. In Massachusetts, 3.7 million patients were studied, and it was shown that 31% of them had visited a minimum of two hospitals in the previous five years [15].
- *Unstructured text*: Even though there are several defined frameworks for data collection, the majority of EHR data is unstructured text. These details are available in the form of explanation and documentation. They are simple to understand for people, but it is challenging to find the correct data using automatic computing approaches. Complex data extraction methods like natural language processing (NLP) are being used to extract knowledge from text notes [16].
- *Selection bias*: The patient population will typically be a random assortment in any institution. It varies according to the type of practice, the care unit, and the institution's location. Demographic variety won't be present. This is a significant obstacle to overcome. Findings from EHR data mining won't be generalizable as a result. While working with the secondary usage of data, this issue must be addressed.
- *Interoperability*: Lack of EHR interoperability is a significant barrier to better healthcare, innovation, and cost reduction. There are several causes for it. Commercially available EHR software comes from closed, proprietary systems. The majority of software was not created to facilitate contact with a third party, and creating novel interfaces for that reason could be expensive. Lack of standards is another factor in the issue. Many patients are not willing to share their information with others. In addition, Health Insurance Portability and Accountability Act (HIPAA Act) [17] compliance is required for EHR systems to guarantee data security and privacy.

2.4 DIFFERENT DATASETS AND TECHNIQUES USED FOR MINING COMORBIDITY PATTERNS IN DIABETIC PATIENTS

Compared to people without diabetes, people with diabetes are more likely to have various illnesses. Comorbidity, which is defined as the occurrence of two or more illnesses in the same individual [18, 19], is of concern for the public health since it has a big impact on both patients and the healthcare system [19, 20]. Numerous studies have found that the comorbidity occurrence varies between approximately 20% and 90% [21–24]. This difference is brought about by the study population as well as additional aspects of the study design, such the comorbidity definition. Comorbidity is more common as people become older and is not just a problem for the elderly [24–27]. With the availability of clinical datasets for data mining, it is possible to identify illness relationships and comorbidity patterns from a patient's clinical history that was gathered over the course of repeated medical care [28–30]. As a result, a lot of academics have looked at comorbidity patterns using clinical data. An overview of the research on mining comorbidity patterns in diabetic patients can be found in Table 2.1.

TABLE 2.1
An overview of the research on mining comorbidity patterns in diabetic patients

Reference	Aim	Dataset	Techniques Used	Remarks
Ahmad Shaker Abdalrada et al. [31]	Prediction of diabetes and cardiovascular disease co-occurrence	Diabetes complications screening research initiative (DiScRi)	Evimp functions, Logistic Regression and classification and regression algorithm	• Found usual risk factors for diabetes and cardiovascular diseases co-occurrence • The forecasting accuracy of the proposed technique is 94.09%, with sensitivity 93.5%, and specificity 95.8% Some limitations: • Dataset has limited coverage of population and time period • Not been tested in a clinical population • Not recorded the run time for the machine learning models
Xueyan Han et al. [32]	Extraction of comorbidity patterns in schizophrenia patients	EHRs from 2015 to 2017 in Beijing, China	Association Rule Mining and Logistic regression analyses	• The five comorbidities that are most prevalent were extracted • Also derived comorbidity combinations linked with daily expense, one-year readmission and length of stay Some limitations: • Dataset has limited coverage of population and time period • Not recorded the run time for the machine learning models
Svetla Boytcheva et al. [33]	Mining comorbidity patterns	Records of outpatient care provided to the Bulgarian National Health Insurance Fund between 2010 and 2016	Frequent pattern mining and text mining	• Some mentioned comorbidities of hyperprolactinemia, schizophrenia and T2D are confirmed • Proposed method can handle large, dense datasets efficiently for trivial relative minimum support values

Author	Topic	Dataset	Methods	Findings / Limitations
				Some limitations: • Sequences of diseases have not explored • Dataset has limited coverage of population and time period • Not recorded the run time for the machine learning models
Piotr Dworzynski et al. [34]	Nationwide prediction of T2D comorbidities	Danish health registers data	Logistic regression, gradient boosting and random forest models	• Demonstrated how to use registry data to routinely locate those at risk of getting disease comorbidities • Also suggested that the use of additional data like lab measurements, genotyping, socio-economic data etc could improve the outcomes Some limitations: • Have not used the temporal dimension in the data • Dataset has limited coverage of population and time period
Magdalena Nowakowska et al. [35]	Quantifying T2D comorbidity patterns	Clinical Practice Research Datalink (CPRD) linked with the Index of Multiple Deprivation (IMD)	Linear regression and hierarchical clustering	• Identified clusters of similar conditions • This is the largest study yet conducted in England on comorbidities in T2D patients Some limitations: • Has not focused on comorbidity progression • Dataset has limited coverage of population and time period • Not recorded the run time for the machine learning models

(continued)

TABLE 2.1 (Continued)
An overview of the research on mining comorbidity patterns in diabetic patients

Reference	Aim	Dataset	Techniques Used	Remarks
Inmaculada Guerrero-Fernández de Alba et al. [36]	Analysing T2D mellitus comorbidity	EHRs from the Information System for Research Development in Primary Care (SIDIAP)	Logistic regression models	• Gives a visual depiction so that anyone with varying interests, including both the general public and health experts can view and investigate the connections between diseases • Additionally, created trajectories that display temporal relationships and indicate the conditions like retinopathy that play a vital role in the T2D development Some limitations: • Dataset has limited coverage of population and time period • Not recorded the run time for the machine learning models
Yifei Wang et al. [37]	Analysing the prevalence and relationships between comorbid conditions in Chinese adult patients with T2D	Chinese patients' data	Association rules and complex network	• Top 10 comorbidities were identified Some limitations: • Dataset has limited coverage of population and time period • The regional factors are not considered in the data analysis • Causality between combined diseases was not analysed and discussed
Hui Chen et al. [38]	Assessing the prevalence and trends of comorbid conditions in adult patients	Data on hospital discharges in Northeast China from 2002 to 2013	Statistical analysis	• Assessed the prevalence of T2D in China, particularly in Northeast China, using huge electronic medical record-derived data • Twenty-seven conditions were identified as important comorbidities of T2D

Hye Soon Kim et al. [39]	Analysing comorbidity in patients with T2D	Patients' data from 1996 to 2007 in Keimyung University Dongsan	Association rule mining	Some limitations: • Dataset has limited coverage of population and time period • Not recorded the time taken by the machine learning models • Revealed associations of comorbidity and found that the key factor in the relationship between T2D and its concomitant illnesses is essential hypertension • Developed Dx Analyse Tool Some limitations: • Dataset has limited coverage of population and time period • Not recorded the run time for the machine learning models • Has not focused on comorbidity progression
Abdelaali Hassaine et al. [40]	Mining disease clusters and their trajectories simultaneously	CPRD	Non-negative matrix factorization (NMF)	• Explored multimorbidity patterns using NMF for temporal phenotyping • Developed a system to assess the efficacy of multimorbidity clusters and trajectories Some limitations: • Have used subjective / arbitrary thresholds • To evaluate if the found relationships are actually meaningful or not, further research is required

(*continued*)

TABLE 2.1 (Continued)
An overview of the research on mining comorbidity patterns in diabetic patients

Reference	Aim	Dataset	Techniques Used	Remarks
Adrian Martinez-De la Torre et al. [41]	Finding frequent comorbidity clusters, then examining how newly treated T2D patients' conditions change over time	IQVIA Medical Research Data (IMRD)	Bayesian nonparametric model	• Among patients with recently treated T2D, clusters of chronic illness comorbidities were discovered • Also found the disease progression patterns Some limitations: • Not taken into account the various degrees of severity that a long-lasting illness might have had • Not included treatments of pharmacological
Otovwe Agofure et al. [42]	Identify the pattern of diabetes mellitus complications and comorbidities	General Hospital Ughelli Delta State, Nigeria	Statistical Analysis	• Showed that the occurrence of heart attack and kidney failure as difficulties and hypertension as a co-occurring disorder in diabetes patients • Also revealed that the female diabetes cases were more compared to male Some limitations: • The study only used one facility; thus, it might not be typical of the overall population and could possibly be subject to selection bias • Dataset has limited coverage of population and time period • Has not focused on comorbidity progression
Mengfei Guo et al. [43]	Analysis of disease comorbidity patterns	453 hospitals across China	Statistical analysis	• Identified clinically meaningful disease comorbidity communities • Additionally, the presence of the disease was predicted using solely the temporal correlations between the disease characteristics

Author	Focus	Dataset	Technique	Observation
				Some limitations: • Dataset has limited coverage of population and time period • Not recorded the run time for the machine learning models
Francesco Folino et al. [44]	Prediction of disease risk	1,462 patients' data of a small town in the south of Italy	Statistical analysis	• Explored a phenotypic comorbidity network • Proposed a prediction model to determine the risk of individuals to develop future diseases Some limitations: • Dataset has limited coverage of population and time period • Has not focused on comorbidity progression • Has not evaluated the proposed model against existing models in the literature
Bramesh S M et al. [45]	Clustering comorbidity patterns of diabetic patients	Clinical datasets	Latent Dirichlet allocation and hierarchical clustering	• Proposed an efficient and scalable technique to cluster the EHR data • Has worked on more than one clinical dataset Some limitations: • Has not focused on comorbidity progression • Not recorded the run time for the machine learning models

For mining comorbidity patterns in diabetes patients, several researchers have explored a variety of strategies in the past, as indicated in Table 2.1. In summary, these techniques can be grouped into pairwise techniques (relative risk, Pearson correlation, observed/expected ratios and so on), statistical techniques (logistic regression, linear regression, Bayesian nonparametric model, and so on), and probabilistic techniques (association rule mining, frequent pattern mining, and so on). The use of these techniques, in our opinion, could be advantageous for those attempting to identify unique comorbidity patterns in diabetes patients from EHR data and could result in new findings or further affirmatory research.

In conclusion, EHRs from the DiScRi, CPRD, SIDIAP, IMRD, and so on provide an opportunity for the researchers to explore comorbidity patterns in diabetic patients. But due to HIPAA laws not all researchers have access to EHRs; on the other hand, incidence of comorbidities in diabetic patients is increasing day by day, so we can say that comorbidity patterns in diabetic patients is not yet completely explored and it needs to be addressed.

2.5 CONCLUSIONS

The future of patient care in medical practices and hospitals will undoubtedly involve electronic health records. This chapter deliberates some aspects of the EHRs. In addition to healthcare advantages like efficient way for information exchange, improved patients' medical records management, safety, reduced costs, improved patient care and enhancing population health in general, it creates a great opening for mining comorbidity patterns in diabetic patients. A patient's quality of life, health condition, outcomes, and hospitalization are all impacted by diabetes and its comorbidities [46–48]. It is significant to highlight that, in 2017, there were 67.9 million disability-adjusted life years linked with diabetes, with a forecast of 79.3 million in 2025 [49]. However, given the disparity between the high frequency of diabetic patients suffering from more than one disease simultaneously and the relatively lower number of research papers [50], which is partially a result of a lack of data due to the significant restrictions on the utilization of EHR data in research purposes, studies on comorbidity are extremely difficult. Finally, this chapter can serve as a helpful tool for researchers when preparing future interventions to investigate comorbidity patterns in diabetic patients.

REFERENCES

[1] Islam, S. M. S., Purnat, T. D., Phuong, N. T. A., Mwingira, U., Schacht, K., & Fröschl, G. (2014). Non-Communicable Diseases (NCDs) in developing countries: a symposium report. *Globalization and Health*, 10(1), 1–8.

[2] Vos, T., Lim, S. S., Abbafati, C., Abbas, K. M., Abbasi, M., Abbasifard, M., & Bhutta, Z. A. (2020). Global burden of 369 diseases and injuries in 204 countries and territories, 1990–2019: a systematic analysis for the Global Burden of Disease Study 2019. *The Lancet*, 396(10258), 1204–1222.

[3] Atlas, D. (2015). *IDF Diabetes Atlas*, 7th edn. Brussels, Belgium: International Diabetes Federation.

[4] Piette, J. D., & Kerr, E. A. (2006). The impact of comorbid chronic conditions on diabetes care. *Diabetes Care*, 29(3), 725–731.
[5] Kim, E., Rubinstein, S., Nead, K., Wojcieszynski, A., Gabriel, P., & Warner, J. (2019). The evolving use of electronic health records (EHR) for research. *Seminars in Radiation Oncology*, 29, 354–361.
[6] Sun, W., Cai, Z., Li, Y., Liu, F., Fang, S., & Wang, G. (2018). Data processing and text mining technologies on electronic medical records: a review. *Journal of Healthcare Engineering*, 2018, 1–9. https://doi.org/10.1155/2018/4302425
[7] https://archive.ics.uci.edu/ml/datasets/diabetes+130-us+hospitals+for+years+1999-2008
[8] Kruse, C. S., Kristof, C., Jones, B., Mitchell, E., & Martinez, A. (2016). Barriers to electronic health record adoption: a systematic literature review. *Journal of Medical Systems*, 40(12), 252. https://doi.org/10.1007/s10916-016-0628-9
[9] Bayley, K. B., Belnap, T., Savitz, L., Masica, A. L., Shah, N., & Fleming, N. S. (2013). Challenges in using electronic health record data for CER: experience of 4 learning organizations and solutions applied. *Medical Care*, 51, S80–S86.
[10] Wu, J., Roy, J., & Stewart, W. F. (2010). Prediction modeling using EHR data: challenges, strategies, and a comparison of machine learning approaches. *Medical Care*, 48(6), S106–S113.
[11] Paxton, C., Niculescu-Mizil, A., & Saria, S. (2013). Developing predictive models using electronic medical records: challenges and pitfalls. In AMIA Annual Symposium Proceedings (Vol. 2013, p. 1109). American Medical Informatics Association.
[12] Wells, B. J., Chagin, K. M., Nowacki, A. S., & Kattan, M. W. (2013). Strategies for handling missing data in electronic health record derived data. *Egems*, 1(3), 1–7.
[13] Hersh, W. *Secondary Use of Clinical Data from Electronic Health Records*. Oregon Health & Science University.
[14] Botsis, T., Hartvigsen, G., Chen, F., & Weng, C. (2010). Secondary use of EHR: data quality issues and informatics opportunities. *Summit on Translational Bioinformatics*, 2010, 1.
[15] Bourgeois, F. C., Olson, K. L., & Mandl, K. D. (2010). Patients treated at multiple acute health care facilities: quantifying information fragmentation. *Archives of Internal Medicine*, 170(22), 1989–1995.
[16] Murff, H. J., FitzHenry, F., Matheny, M. E., Gentry, N., Kotter, K. L., Crimin, K., ... & Speroff, T. (2011). Automated identification of postoperative complications within an electronic medical record using natural language processing. *Jama*, 306(8), 848–855.
[17] Act, A. (1996). Health insurance portability and accountability act of 1996. *Public Law*, 104, 191.
[18] Van den A. M., B. F., & Knottnerus, J. A. (1996). Comorbidity or multimorbidity. *European Journal of General Practice*, 2(2), 65–70.
[19] Valderas, J. M., Starfield, B., Sibbald, B., Salisbury, C., & Roland, M. (2009). Defining comorbidity: implications for understanding health and health services. *The Annals of Family Medicine*, 7(4), 357–363.
[20] Gijsen, R., Hoeymans, N., Schellevis, F. G., Ruwaard, D., Satariano, W. A., & van den Bos, G. A. (2001). Causes and consequences of comorbidity: a review. *Journal of Clinical Epidemiology*, 54(7), 661–674.
[21] Bonavita, V., & De Simone, R. (2008). Towards a definition of comorbidity in the light of clinical complexity. *Neurological Sciences*, 29(1), 99–102.
[22] Fortin, M., Lapointe, L., Hudon, C., & Vanasse, A. (2005). Multimorbidity is common to family practice: is it commonly researched? *Canadian Family Physician*, 51(2), 244–245.

[23] Mezzich, J. E., & Salloum, I. M. (2008). Clinical complexity and person-centered integrative diagnosis. *World Psychiatry*, 7(1), 1.

[24] Marengoni, A., Angleman, S., Melis, R., Mangialasche, F., Karp, A., Garmen, A., & Fratiglioni, L. (2011). Aging with multimorbidity: a systematic review of the literature. *Ageing Research Reviews*, 10(4), 430–439.

[25] Doshi-Velez, F., Ge, Y., & Kohane, I. (2014). Comorbidity clusters in autism spectrum disorders: an electronic health record time-series analysis. *Pediatrics*, 133(1), e54–e63.

[26] Jakovljevic, M., & Ostojic, L. (2013). Comorbidity and multimorbidity in medicine today: challenges and opportunities for bringing separated branches of medicine closer to each other. *PsychiatrDanub*, 25 (Suppl 1), 18–28.

[27] Taylor, A. W., Price, K., Gill, T. K., Adams, R., Pilkington, R., Carrangis, N., & Wilson, D. (2010). Multimorbidity-not just an older person's issue. Results from an Australian biomedical study. *BMC Public Health*, 10(1), 1–10.

[28] Backenroth, D., Chase, H., Friedman, C., & Wei, Y. (2016). Using rich data on comorbidities in case-control study design with electronic health record data improves control of confounding in the detection of adverse drug reactions. *PLoS One*, 11(10), e0164304.

[29] Bagley, S. C., Sirota, M., Chen, R., Butte, A. J., & Altman, R. B. (2016). Constraints on biological mechanism from disease comorbidity using electronic medical records and database of genetic variants. *PLoS Computational Biology*, 12(4), e1004885.

[30] Holmes, A. B., Hawson, A., Liu, F., Friedman, C., Khiabanian, H., & Rabadan, R. (2011). Discovering disease associations by integrating electronic clinical data and medical literature. *PLoS One*, 6(6), e21132.

[31] Abdalrada, A. S., Abawajy, J., Al-Quraishi, T., & Islam, S. M. S. (2022). Machine learning models for prediction of co-occurrence of diabetes and cardiovascular diseases: a retrospective cohort study. *Journal of Diabetes & Metabolic Disorders*, 21(1), 1–11.

[32] Han, X., Jiang, F., Needleman, J., Zhou, H., Yao, C., & Tang, Y. L. (2022). Comorbidity combinations in schizophrenia inpatients and their associations with service utilization: a medical record-based analysis using association rule mining. *Asian Journal of Psychiatry*, 67, 102927.

[33] Boytcheva, S., Angelova, G., Angelov, Z., & Tcharaktchiev, D. (2017). Mining comorbidity patterns using retrospective analysis of big collection of outpatient records. *Health Information Science and Systems*, 5(1), 1–9.

[34] Dworzynski, P., Aasbrenn, M., Rostgaard, K., Melbye, M., Gerds, T. A., Hjalgrim, H., & Pers, T. H. (2020). Nationwide prediction of type 2 diabetes comorbidities. *Scientific Reports*, 10(1), 1–13.

[35] Nowakowska, M., Zghebi, S. S., Ashcroft, D. M., Buchan, I., Chew-Graham, C., Holt, T., ... & Kontopantelis, E. (2019). The comorbidity burden of type 2 diabetes mellitus: patterns, clusters and predictions from a large English primary care cohort. *BMC Medicine*, 17(1), 1–10.

[36] Guerrero-Fernández de Alba, I., Orlando, V., Monetti, V. M., Mucherino, S., Gimeno-Miguel, A., Vaccaro, O., ... & Menditto, E. (2020). Comorbidity in an older population with type-2 diabetes mellitus: identification of the characteristics and healthcare utilization of high-cost Patients. *Frontiers in Pharmacology*, 11, 586187.

[37] Wang, Y., Xing, Y., Pi, M., Zhang, R., He, X., Zhou, X., ... & Wen, T. (2020, December). Analysis of diabetic comorbidities and their interrelationships in 5227 Chinese patients with type 2 diabetes. In 2020 IEEE International Conference on Bioinformatics and Biomedicine (BIBM) (pp. 1602–1607). IEEE.

[38] Chen, H., Zhang, Y., Wu, D., Gong, C., Pan, Q., Dong, X., ... & Xu, H. (2016). Comorbidity in adult patients hospitalized with type 2 diabetes in Northeast China: an analysis of hospital discharge data from 2002 to 2013. *BioMed Research International*, 2016.

[39] Kim, H. S., Shin, A. M., Kim, M. K., & Kim, Y. N. (2012). Comorbidity study on type 2 diabetes mellitus using data mining. *The Korean Journal of Internal Medicine*, 27(2), 197.

[40] Hassaine, A., Canoy, D., Solares, J. R. A., Zhu, Y., Rao, S., Li, Y., ... & Salimi-Khorshidi, G. (2020). Learning multimorbidity patterns from electronic health records using non-negative matrix factorisation. *Journal of Biomedical Informatics*, 112, 103606.

[41] Martinez-De la Torre, A., Perez-Cruz, F., Weiler, S., & Burden, A. M. (2022). Comorbidity clusters associated with newly treated Type 2 diabetes mellitus: a Bayesian nonparametric analysis. medRxiv. https://doi.org/10.1101/2022.04.07.22273569

[42] Agofure, O., Okandeji-Barry, O. R., & Ogbon, P. (2020). Pattern of diabetes mellitus complications and co-morbidities in Ughelli north local government area, Delta State, Nigeria. *Nigerian Journal of Basic and Clinical Sciences*, 17(2), 123.

[43] Guo, M., Yu, Y., Wen, T., Zhang, X., Liu, B., Zhang, J., ... & Zhou, X. (2019). Analysis of disease comorbidity patterns in a large-scale China population. *BMC Medical Genomics*, 12(12), 1–10.

[44] Folino, F., Pizzuti, C., & Ventura, M. (2010, September). A comorbidity network approach to predict disease risk. In International Conference on Information Technology in Bio-and Medical Informatics (pp. 102–109). Springer, Berlin, Heidelberg.

[45] Bramesh, S. M., & Anil Kumar, K. M. (2022). An efficient and scalable technique for clustering comorbidity patterns of diabetic patients from clinical datasets. *International Journal of Modern Education and Computer Science* (IJMECS), 14(6), 35–52. DOI:10.5815/ijmecs.2022.06.04

[46] Zghebi, S. S., Steinke, D. T., Rutter, M. K., & Ashcroft, D. M. (2020). Eleven-year multimorbidity burden among 637 255 people with and without type 2 diabetes: a population-based study using primary care and linked hospitalisation data. *BMJ Open*, 10(7), e033866.

[47] Argano, C., Natoli, G., Mularo, S., Nobili, A., Monaco, M. L., Mannucci, P. M., ... & Corrao, S. (2022, January). Impact of diabetes mellitus and its comorbidities on elderly patients hospitalized in internal medicine wards: data from the RePoSi registry. *Healthcare* 10(1), 86.

[48] Nowakowska, M., Zghebi, S. S., Ashcroft, D. M., Buchan, I., Chew-Graham, C., Holt, T., ... & Kontopantelis, E. (2020). Correction to: the comorbidity burden of type 2 diabetes mellitus: patterns, clusters and predictions from a large English primary care cohort. *BMC Medicine*, 18(1), 22. doi: 10.1186/s12916-020-1492-5

[49] Lin, X., Xu, Y., Pan, X., Xu, J., Ding, Y., Sun, X., ... & Shan, P. F. (2020). Global, regional, and national burden and trend of diabetes in 195 countries and territories: an analysis from 1990 to 2025. *Scientific Reports*, 10(1), 1–11.

[50] Xu, X., Mishra, G. D., & Jones, M. (2017). Mapping the global research landscape and knowledge gaps on multimorbidity: a bibliometric study. *Journal of Global Health*, 7(1). doi: 10.7189/jogh.07.010414

3 Fundamentals and Technicalities of Big Data and Analytics

Partha Ghosh, Ananya Biswas and Suradhuni Ghosh

3.1 INTRODUCTION

Our daily decisions are driven by information and data, which are then used as fuel by capable explanatory computations to create a more intelligent and productive environment. We all deserve more. This underutilised area of technology has been categorised as Big Data and analytics, and both the academic and technical communities see it as a competitive innovation with the potential to create important untapped riches and opportunities.

Since the 1990s, people have been referring to huge information as "big data," and some people attribute this to John Mashey. When businesses first started utilising computers to store and analyse massive volumes of data, as more frequently resorted to computers to aid in making sense of the exponentially growing volumes of data created by their operations, big data started to take off.

In or around 2005, people started to realise how much data users were generating through Facebook, YouTube, and other web platforms. The introduction of Hadoop, an open-source system created largely to store and analyse massive data volumes, occurred in the same year.

We may anticipate seeing even more incredible and revolutionary uses for this technology in the years to come as the discipline of big data analytics continues to develop. Since then, the amount of big data has exponentially increased.

Every day, terabytes of data are generated from sources such as social media, company information, financials, and customer intelligence, as well as trade sensors and electronic devices like as smart phones and automobiles.

Volume, velocity, veracity, and variety are the primary characteristics that define data as Big Data.

Big data is defined as collections of datasets so large in dimensions that traditional databases (Oracle, SAP) and data processing tools face challenges to store, manage, process, and analyse the data.

In recent times, there has been an exponential rise in the amount of structured, unstructured, and semi-structured data generated by data innovation, mechanical, healthcare, retail, web, and diverse frameworks, which is still ongoing. As the volume grows, parallel processing and a unique storage approach are required for Big Data, which necessitates the use of many, typically thousands, of machines.

Massive data analysis makes use of cutting-edge tools and techniques (like Hadoop, Apache Spark, and Scala) to extract meaningful information and insights from massive data sets. The process of gathering this information from many sources, organising it for advance ingestion, analysing it, and ultimately making it available to the end user is referred to as big data architecture.

Big Data enables businesses to make better decisions, reduce business process costs, detect fraud, increase productivity, improve customer service, and boost business agility. Some good-to-known technologies of Big Data include predictive analytics, NoSQL databases, knowledge discovery tools, stream analytics, distributed storage, data integration, and data pre-processing.

Thus, big data and analytics refer to the collection, storage, processing, and analysis of massive amounts of data on cloud-based computing systems. The potential uses of big data have been further increased by cloud computing. To test a portion of data, developers may quickly put up ad-hoc clusters in the cloud, thanks to its true elastic scalability.

Every second, the volume of healthcare data is growing larger, making it more difficult to find any useful information. The demand for healthcare has risen rapidly, necessitating a greater emphasis on healthcare management and innovative medicines. This demand has been the driving force behind the development of new technologies in the healthcare industry.

Recent advances in big data analytics have changed outdated techniques for gathering data into insightful understandings. This benefits the healthcare industry in many ways, including the potential to identify life-threatening illnesses early and deliver better treatment to the right individuals at the right time, improving the bar for patient care. For the evaluation and integration of enormous volumes of extremely critical structured, semi-structured, and unstructured data generated quickly from clinical, hospital, social web, and health data lakes. The use of enormous data analytics within the healthcare business is one of the most important concerns that may arise over the next several years, according to International Data Corporation (IDC).

According to IDC, big data with a slew of tools will have a massive impact on the healthcare industry when compared to other industries. These tools will collect, manage, analyse, and assimilate massive amounts of data generated by today's healthcare system. A few numbers of applications of big data are shown in Figure 3.1.

Regardless, this chapter discusses a few concerns of contemporary health information analytics stages that provide specific tools for data collecting, aggregation, management, investigation, visualisation, and translation.

This chapter will provide a brief overview of the definition, characteristics, types, components, benefits, big data analytical tools and technologies, and most recent insights of big data. The various stages of the healthcare industry from data collection to data delivery are examined in this chapter. The road map of big medical data processing are shown in Figure 3.2.

Fundamentals and Technicalities of Big Data and Analytics

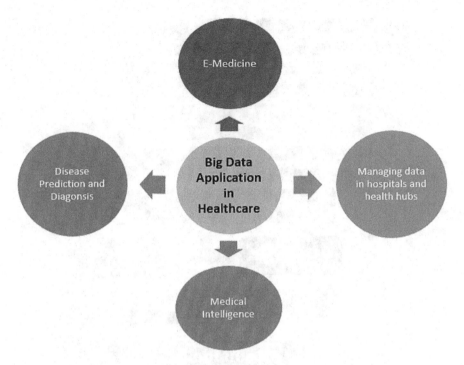

FIGURE 3.1 Big data application in healthcare.

In addition, a concise case study using MapReduce tool has been discussed in depth to demonstrate the significant impact on diabetes disease identification and diagnosis. This will provide a better understanding about the application of big data in the healthcare system.

3.2 WHAT IS BIG DATA?

Big data is just a more extensive, sophisticated collection of data that has been gathered from various, both new and old sources. Large, varied data sets that are expanding at an exponential rate are referred to as big data. It is a massive collection of data that keeps expanding over time. As the data sets are so large, conventional data processing software is unable to handle them. These enormous amounts of data are typically employed to solve business challenges that you might not be able to handle.

As the name suggests, it alludes to sophisticated knowledge sets that need to be processed and analysed in order to find crucial information that can help enterprises and organisations. Big data is an assortment of organised, semi-structured, and unstructured data that is produced by enterprises and may be used for advanced analytics jobs like machine learning projects, prognostic modelling, and other things.

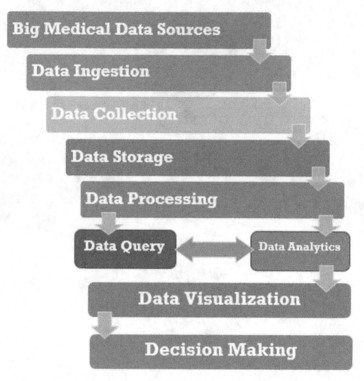

FIGURE 3.2 Roadmap of big medical data processing.

Big data is often characterised by the three V's:

- the significant *volume* of data in many situations;
- the large *variety* of data types that are often stored in big data systems; and
- A measure of how quickly data is produced, gathered, and interpreted, that is, *velocity*.

Doug Laney first noted these traits in 2001. Veracity, value, and variability are a few more V's that have lately been added to various definitions of big data.

The term big data is used to describe data sets that are too large or too different in type to be captured, managed, and processed by conventional relational databases in a low-latency manner. Therefore, big data has one or more of the following traits: high volume, high velocity, or high variety.

New types and sources of data are increasing the complexity of data, driven by artificial intelligence (AI), mobile devices, social media, and the Internet of Things (IoT). For example, big data comes from sensors, devices, video/audio, networks, log files, transactional applications, the web, and social media, much of it real-time and at scale.

Businesses, government organisations, healthcare providers, financial institutions, and academic institutions are all using the potential of big data to improve consumer experiences and business possibilities. Along with the aforementioned instances, the following list includes some major big data sources:

- *Social media*: Twitter, YouTube, Instagram, Facebook, WhatsApp. Every action you take on these platforms, such as uploading a photo or video, messaging someone, leaving a comment, pressing "like," etc., creates data.
- *A sensor placed in various places*: A sensor that collects information on temperature, humidity, etc. is put around the city. By placing a camera alongside the road, traffic data is collected and stored. A lot of data is produced by security cameras installed in high-traffic locations like airports, train stations, and shopping centres.
- *Customer satisfaction feedback*: Data is generated by customer reviews posted on a company's website regarding their goods or services. For instance, retail commercial websites like Amazon, Walmart, Flipkart, and Myntra collect consumer feedback on the calibre of their offering and turnaround time. Other service-providing businesses like telecoms aim to improve client satisfaction. They generate a great deal of data.
- *IoT appliances*: Smart TVs, washing machines, coffee makers, air conditioners, and other connected electronic gadgets generate data for their smart functionality. These data are produced by machines using sensors that are housed in various devices.
- *E-commerce*: Many saved records are regarded as one of the sources of big data in e-commerce transactions, corporate transactions, banking, and the stock market. Payments made via debit or credit cards or other electronic methods are all kept on file as data.
- *Global positioning system* (GPS): The GPS in the car aids in tracking its movement to reduce the distance travelled and the amount of time needed to get there. Huge amounts of data about vehicle position and motion are produced by this technology.

Applications of big data in the healthcare sector are rapidly expanding in the modern day, and their significance is highlighted here.

3.3 WHY IS BIG DATA CRUCIAL TO THE HEALTHCARE INDUSTRY?

Organisations will use big data, for example, in the medical field. Big data is also utilised in the medical industry to identify disease risk factors and by clinicians to assist in the creation of diagnosis for their patients' maladies.

Medical researchers use it to look for disease signs and risk factors, while physicians use it to help diagnose patients' illnesses and medical conditions. A combination of information from electronic health records, social media platforms, the web, and other sources keeps health care organisations and government agencies up to speed on infectious disease threats or outbreaks.

3.4 WHAT IS BIG DATA ANALYTICS?

Only a small part of the data produced by the billions of digital solutions is processed. Companies are now encumbered with data silos due to the infiltration of data into traditional systems. To fully utilise the potential of vast amounts of information, big data analytics must be used at scale in this situation.

Big data analytics looks at a lot of data to find hidden patterns, interconnections, market trends, customer preferences, and other facts. With today's technology, it is feasible to assess our data and obtain responses from it very instantaneously.

Additionally, it speeds up processing to enable firms to make ground-breaking business decisions and makes handling enormous amounts of data easier. The methods, tools, and applications created especially for big data analysis come into play because conventional types of data analysis software are not able to support this degree of complexity and scale. Big data analytics is the application of cutting-edge analytical methods to very large, diversified data sets that contain a variety of data kinds from numerous sources, ranging from terabytes to zettabytes.

Four categories of big data analytics exist: diagnostic, descriptive, prescriptive, and predictive. To improve the process of information research and ensure that the organisation benefits from the information they receive, they utilise a number of technologies for activities like information mining, cleansing, integration, representation, and many others.

- *Descriptive analysis*, which shows what has already occurred
- *Diagnostic analysis*, which aims to comprehend the reasons behind events
- *Predictive analysis*, which uses historical data to identify trends for the future
- *Prescriptive analysis*, which enables you to offer suggestions for the future.

Healthcare-related data, including persistent records, well-being plans, protections data, and other types of data, are difficult to manage but are packed with valuable insights that can be gleaned once analytics are coupled.

Big data analytics are essential to the healthcare industry for this reason.

Healthcare professionals can almost instantly offer life-saving diagnosis or treatment alternatives by speedily analysing massive amounts of structured and unstructured data.

Since we now know what big data and its analytics are, let's go over the different types of big data.

3.5 BIG DATA TYPES IN HEALTHCARE

Numerous healthcare sources provide enormous amounts of data. It is challenging to combine this enormous amount of data into a system since it is so diverse in terms of format, type, and context. A data scientist's main goal is to uncover hidden patterns in information collected from multiple sources in an exceedingly extremely effective manner that may be simply modified for the patient's higher care. Figure 3.3 displays the potential big data sources that could be employed in healthcare.

Fundamentals and Technicalities of Big Data and Analytics

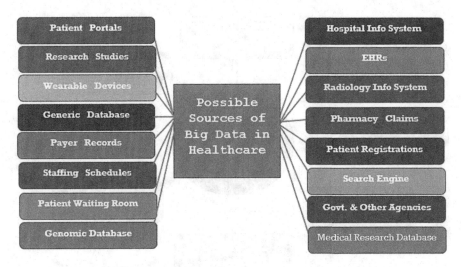

FIGURE 3.3 All possible big data sources in healthcare.

TABLE 3.1
Example of structured data in a hospital

Patient ID	Patient Name	Doctor Name	Department
1001	Partha Ghosh	Dr. Saktipada Ghosh	Paediatrics
1002	Suradhuni Ghosh	Dr. A. R. Ghosh	Gynaecology
1003	Ananya Biswas	Dr. G. P. Biswas	Endocrinology

3.5.1 STRUCTURED DATA

Structured data is prepared using a predetermined outline and is arranged in a tabular format. The data is grabbed and stored in discrete coded values in this instance. A connection is kept between each column in the structured data. For a data manager in a healthcare institution, computation and analysis are made simpler by structured data storage.

In the fields of diagnosis, laboratories, and pharmaceuticals, structured datasets are given emphasis. Some patients, for example, have a clinic agreement with a specialist. As shown in Table 3.1, the electronic recording frameworks can be created. Table 3.1 serves as an illustration of how structured data is applied in a hospital.

3.5.2 UNSTRUCTURED DATA

Unstructured data lacks a standard format. It doesn't have any set boundaries. It is incompatible with relational databases like structured databases. Eighty percent of the world's information volume is present there. Text is one sort of unstructured data, although other non-text data also behaves like the unstructured type.

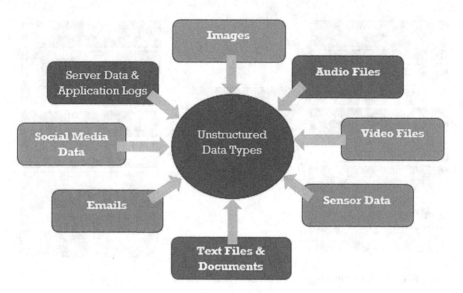

FIGURE 3.4 Possible unstructured data types.

Images and video are two types of unstructured non-text data. The majority of healthcare business emails, patient registration forms, survey replies, radiographic pictures, audible sounds, and other documents contain unstructured data.

The biomedical industry is where you'll find the majority of text-based unstructured data. Both structured and unstructured data must be analysed when using big data analytics. Figure 3.4 displays a number of potential unstructured data formats.

3.5.3 Semi-structured Data

One must work with a semi-structured database if they want the benefit from both the structured and unstructured data. Tabular semi-structured data is not an immutable component of any rational database, but it does have several significant qualities that facilitate examination.

Semi-structured data includes formats like NoSQL, electronic data interchange (EDI), and others. Although certain free-text and hierarchically arranged collections of data are created by semi-structured databases, there are no restrictions on how much data a data processor might choose to keep.

3.5.4 Genomic Data

The dataset that pertains to the DNA and genome of a living organism contains genomic data. In the healthcare industry, genomic data is generated, processed, and mined using contemporary genomic technology. Computational genomic annotation is referred to as genome data mining. Sequencing, sorting, and assembly of the large genomic data are done using a variety of techniques and software. Healthcare uses a vast amount of genomic and DNA data. To process the structure and functionalities of genome data, sophisticated bioinformatics software is required.

3.5.5 Sentiment Data

In the current state of healthcare, medical sentiment analysis is a relatively new and alarming problem. Patients and their families are interested in learning about the most recent medical advancements and facility evaluations for specific physicians, hospitals, or diagnostic centres. A conventional method of questions and responses is the most effective technique to gather this data [1]. In this approach, patients and their loved ones question people they know who may have visited a hospital or other healthcare facility. On several social media sites, this commentary can be found. One illustration is that one can find these insightful reviews on a blog article. Sentiment analysis is a field that classifies opinions, remarks, or thoughts into two fundamental and intrinsic emotional indications, namely positive and negative [2]. Sentiment analysis refers to the comprehension of the emotional underpinnings of any text and the evaluation of the nature of the text's opinions. The main sources for medical sentiment analysis research are electronic medical records (EMRs) and biomedical literature.

Several studies have recently attempted to collect the medical texts from social media in various medical contexts. Radiology reports, nursing letters, and hospital discharge forms were prepared by the researchers and imported from the MIMIC II database [3]. They also gathered medicine reviews from physician websites like WebMD and Drug Rating.

3.5.6 Clinical Data

A cloud platform is used to compile clinical data, which includes information about patient diagnoses, exposures, demographics, test results, and family links. The majority of clinical information is gathered from patient treatment plans that are still in effect.

Clinical data includes things like electronic health records, patient registries, claims data, health surveys, administrative data, and results from clinical trials. An electronic medical record-keeping system can be used to gather administrative and demographic information, physiological status monitoring for patients, drug prescriptions, patient insurance, and more. EMR is a fantastic source of a fair amount of data, as was already mentioned. Various chronic illnesses, including heart disease, cancer, asthma, Alzheimer's disease, and others, can be monitored for the registered patient.

The National Program of Cancer Registries, Global Alzheimer's Association Interactive Network (GAAIN), National Trauma Data Bank, and National Cardiovascular Data Registry (NCDR) are among well-known databanks for these types of chronic disorders.

We must become familiar with the fundamental aspects of big data if you want to comprehend it effectively. We shall talk about Big Data characteristics in the part after this.

3.6 HEALTHCARE-RELATED BIG DATA CHARACTERISTICS

Big data is typically described using phrases that begin with the letter "v." The three V's—volume, variety, and velocity—were first articulated in 2001 by Doug Laney, a former Gartner analyst who is now a consultant with West Monroe. Today, a longer list of V's with some characteristics is frequently used to characterise big data. The development of V's and big data characteristics in healthcare applications are discussed in this section. The characteristics of large health data are generally related to several difficulties, such as data collection, cleaning, integration, storage, processing, indexing, search, sharing, transfer, mining, analysis, and visualisation.

Numerous researchers have received recommendations for a wide range of V's including volume, diversity, velocity, veracity, and validity for various uses at various times. In order to do effective big data analytics, other academics also predicted [4] that it will soon be increased to 100 V. The following is a summary of some other significant big data characteristics for the healthcare application:

3.6.1 Volume

Big data is extremely large; precisely, it is both uncountable and unmanageable in quantity. Large amounts of data can be ingested, processed, and stored using big data in the healthcare industry. Big healthcare data does not have a predetermined cut off point. Healthcare data in the United States has already surpassed 150 exabytes (10^{18}) nine years ago. For a country like China or India with a large inhabitants, we are dealing with data sizes of zettabyte (10^{21}) and yottabyte (10^{23}).

Every minute, YouTube receives around 500 hours of new video. According to research, 90% of the world's data has just been created in the last two years, and in 2020, roughly 1.7 MB of data are produced per second by each individual [5].

3.6.1.1 Effect of Growing Healthcare Data Volume

Technology development and a continuously growing population have led to an unprecedented increase in health data in recent years. Nearly 30% of all daily data is produced by the healthcare sector, according to RBC Capital Markets. This number is projected to grow, outpacing many other big businesses and giving researchers and analysts access to enormous amounts of data. Data from one patient can fill several megabytes of storage space thanks to the development of increasingly potent diagnostic technologies. This vast amount of data has stimulated new research and made it possible to analyse diseases and treatments in greater depth. It enables a more scientific method of issue solving. Data collection from various healthcare delivery phases in proper time has improved hospital management and patient care.

3.6.2 Velocity

The rate of increase and frequency of supply of data are referred as velocity. The primary cause of healthcare data's exponential growth is velocity. Gigantic amounts of data are being generated; hence high-speed solutions like streaming analytics are frequently used. As users interact with the system in real time, data is recorded. Others might be assembled in groups and spoken out briefly. The back-end of an organisation needs to be effective at handling and storing this data.

3.6.2.1 Effect of Increased Data Velocity in Healthcare

The amount of healthcare-related data has increased, and it is being produced at an astronomically rapid rate. Data generation is accelerating along with studies into data collection and use. As IoT-based healthcare solutions proliferate globally, data-generating processes like these are producing data at higher rates. In 2020 only, data velocity has significantly increased as a result of enhanced data collection methods and a spike in interest in data analysis. This has compelled the industry to create new and better ways to retain and use this data while maintaining patient privacy. Information must be delivered from the source to the destination in the shortest amount of time possible at the time of treatment.

3.6.3 VARIETY

The variety of data is one of the characteristics in big data processing. Data may be communicated and stored in a variety of formats thanks to technology advancement. *Excel* and *CSV* were the only two file types that were commonly used in the past. The forms of data that can now be used include XML, JSON, photos, videos, and many others. Though this variety is helpful in accurately portraying data, caution must be used when combining data from various sources and making sure that systems are capable of comprehending newer forms.

3.6.3.1 Effect of Variety in Healthcare Data

Testing, diagnosis, surgery, monitoring, and long-term care all contribute to the data. Health records, in particular, contain x-rays, lab findings, patient records, CT scans, patient vitals, and so on.

One problem that many organisations ran into while trying to use a wide range of data is lack uniformity among the various sources. Different nations may have different laws regarding the handling, storing, and inconsistent structure of data. Therefore, big data in healthcare is produced from a variety of sources.

These data contain a mixture of organised and unstructured data. Unstructured data complicates data mining and storage. Combining different sources of freely available biological information yields informational heterogeneity and variation in healthcare. The healthcare sector produces data that is based on text, audio, video, and images.

3.6.4 VALUE

Not all data is valuable. We must extract the potential information from the big healthcare dataset. Value is the translation of data with importance. Based on its worth, a data scientist chooses whether to keep or discard data. If the data is not relevant for further processing, there is no need to preserve it, as this consumes storage space and raises storage costs.

3.6.4.1 Effect of Value on Healthcare Data

Use analytical techniques and tools to glean important information from medical records. For instance, this form of analysis helps medical professionals to get fresh insights and provide patients with increasing value as more data becomes available. Additionally, the patients' judgements decide the true value, and occasionally the sum of the information has different values that will increase risk.

3.6.5 Veracity

Recognising the pertinence of information is the key to determining value. The authenticity of data is often described in terms of bias, noise, and irregularity. A data scientist needs to be able to use pertinent information to accomplish their objectives. It is useless to analyse missing data. The veracity requires the collection of a substantial amount of data from many sources. The data processor should make an effort to increase the data set's signal-to-noise ratio. If the dataset is not initially cleaned, veracity suffers.

3.6.5.1 Effects of Data Veracity in the Healthcare Sector

This refers to the demand for an upfront assessment of how trustworthy and accurate particular data sets are in healthcare. Thus, the authenticity of medical data is defined as its accuracy. Due to the fact that poor veracity can drastically lower the accuracy of conclusions, it is one of the most important components of big data.

3.6.6 Variability

It is about establishing whether the data flow's contextualisation structure is trustworthy and enduring even under very unstable circumstances. It explains the need to compile important data while taking into account all probable conditions.

3.6.6.1 Effect of Variability in Healthcare Data

The health-related information gathered from various data sources is updated at various intervals of time. Consistency will also grow in the context of delivering unexpected, concealed, and useful information as the variability of the data changes amid handling and life cycle.

3.6.7 Validity

Validity measures how accurate and true the data is for the purpose for which it is being used, much like veracity does. Validity is now required because of the current rise in privacy concerns. This refers to whether the source was reliable or if it was linked to the appropriate IDs or individuals.

A clinical trial's findings, for instance, may be relevant to a patient's disease symptoms in the context of healthcare. However, the outcomes of a clinical trial cannot be accepted at face value by a doctor treating that patient.

Veracity and validity share certain commonalities. The term "validity" refers to how accurate big data is for a certain purpose, as its definition says. Interestingly, a sizable amount of large data is still useless and is referred to as "dark data."

3.6.8 Volatility

Big data changes constantly. It's possible that the knowledge you learned from a source yesterday differs from what you learned today. Your data's homogeneity is impacted by this phenomenon, which is referred to as data volatility.

3.6.9 Visualisation

Visualisation is the representation of insights from big data in the form of visual materials such as charts and graphs. As big data experts often share their knowledge with non-technical audiences, this has become more common recently.

The extensive application of data analytics has maybe had the greatest effect on the medical field. From identification to therapy, it is employed in a variety of ways at every level [6]. Experts can now more quickly track and predict illnesses thanks to analytics, which also makes it possible to effectively stop the spread. Hospital data and demographic statistics allow for rapid diagnosis and eradication of epidemics. Predictive algorithms support a more accurate diagnosis in difficult situations. The COVID-19 outbreak was being tracked by a number of organisations and companies using real-time data. The process of identifying high-risk patients has been used with it [7]. Additionally, it is utilised in clinical monitoring, where sensors and IoT technology are integrated to track a patient's vital signs.

Smarter homes are now possible because to the development of cloud computing and Internet of Things (IoT) technology. Technologies that have been shown to be more energy efficient include automated lighting and sensor-based temperature controllers. Adoption of greener technologies has become more widespread thanks to data analytics [8]. With the widespread use of 5G technology, the applications for information analytics are as it were anticipated to grow [6].

3.7 ADVANTAGES OF BIG DATA (FEATURES)

- One of the most important benefits of having a lot of data is predictive analytics. Big Data analytics solutions can accurately forecast results, enabling businesses and organisations to make better decisions while streamlining operations and lowering risk.
- Businesses all around the world are improving their effective advertising techniques to raise overall client involvement by utilising data from social media platforms and Big Data analytics tools. Big Data helps organisations improve their products and services by providing insights into the issues that customers are facing.

- To produce highly actionable insights, big data accurately combines pertinent information from several sources. Nearly 43% of firms [9] do not have the necessary tools to get rid of unnecessary data and sort through the clutter to find crucial information. Big data solutions can assist you in minimising this while also helping you save time and money.
- Big Data analytics can assist firms in generating more leads, which will automatically lead to more income. Big data analytics technologies are used by businesses to assess the efficacy of their products and services in terms of consumer and sales. They are then better able to allocate their time and resources.
- You can always stay one step ahead of your competitors by leveraging Big Data experiences. You can conduct market research to see what promos and bargains your competitors are offering in order to better serve your clients. Additionally, you may analyse customer patterns and behaviour using big data insights to provide them with a highly "personalised" experience.

3.8 WHY ARE BIG DATA ANALYTICS CRUCIAL?

Big data analytics enables businesses to use their data to find new opportunities. As a result, the business makes wiser decisions and runs more effectively, which boosts sales and creates happy consumers. As shown in Figure 3.5, businesses employing big data and advanced analytics are providing services in a variety of ways, such as:

- *Cost-cutting measures*. Big data technology, such as cloud-based analytics, can drastically cut expenses when storing massive amounts of data (such as a data lake). A further benefit of big data analytics is that it helps businesses find new, more effective methods to run their operations.
- *Improve decision-making speed*. Businesses can quickly analyse data and make quick, informed decisions thanks to in-memory analytics' speed and flexibility in exploring new data sources, such as streaming data from the Internet of Things.

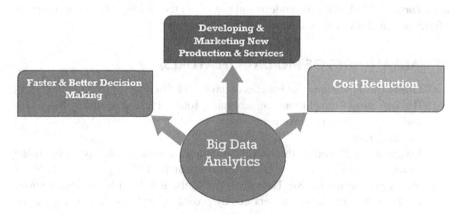

FIGURE 3.5 Businesses that employ big data and sophisticated analytics.

- *Developing and marketing new products and services.* Because businesses can use analytics to determine what customers need and how satisfied they are, they can provide them what they want when they need it. Thanks to big data analytics, more companies have the opportunity to develop innovative new products in response to the changing needs of their customers.

3.9 WHO MAKES USE OF BIG DATA?

Big Data's definition is better understood by those who use it. Consider a few examples of these sectors:

3.9.1 Healthcare

Massive information has already had a significant impact on the healthcare industry. Healthcare professionals (HCP) have made individualised healthcare possible for individual patients through the use of predictive analytics. In addition, Big Data and AI-driven innovations in telemedicine, tele-health, and remote monitoring are enhancing people's lives.

3.9.2 Academia

Big Data is currently improving education as well. There are many online educational courses available, so learning is no longer restricted to the walls of the traditional classroom. To support the holistic development of aspiring students, academic institutions are investing in digital courses backed by Big Data technology.

3.9.3 Banking

Big data is used in the banking business to spot fraud. Big Data solutions are effective in identifying real-time fraud, which includes misusing credit or debit cards, archiving audit trails, manipulating customer statistics improperly, etc.

3.9.4 Manufacturing

According to the TCS Global Trend Study, the two biggest benefits of big data in manufacturing are improved supply strategy and product quality. Industrial big data helps create a transparent infrastructure that anticipates risks and inefficiencies that can negatively impact business operations.

3.9.5 IT

IT organisations are among the world's largest users of big data, using it to improve operations, increase staff productivity, and reduce business risks. The IT sector always supports innovation to handle even the most complicated challenges by combining big data technologies with ML and artificial intelligence.

3.9.5.1 Retail

Big data has altered the way traditional physical stores work. Retailers have amassed massive volumes of data over the years from sources such as neighbourhood demographic surveys, POS scanners, RFID, loyalty cards, in-store inventory, and other sources.

In order to better serve customers, increase sales, and increase revenue, they are now starting to customise the experiences they offer to them. Retailers are already using Wi-Fi and smart sensors to analyse customer movement, the busiest aisles, and how long people spend in them. They also collect data from social media in order to understand what customers are saying about their products and services, which allows them to modify product designs and marketing strategies as needed.

3.9.5.2 Transportation

The transportation industry can benefit greatly from big data analytics. Both private and publicly funded transportation companies use extensive information technologies to improve route planning, coordinate operations, reduce congestion, and improve management in many countries. In addition, the transportation sector uses big data to control revenues, advance technology, enhance logistics, and, of course, dominate the market.

3.10 INSTANCES AND USES OF BIG DATA ANALYTICS IN THE BUSINESS

Here are some instances of how businesses might benefit from big data analytics:

- *Customer acquisition and retention.* Businesses that use trends based on consumer data in their marketing initiatives might boost customer satisfaction. For instance, Spotify, Netflix, and Amazon's personalisation features can improve user experiences and encourage user loyalty.
- *Advertisements were the primary focus.* Clients benefit from engaging targeted marketing campaigns that are tailored to them on a more personal and common level, employing personalisation data from sources such as previous purchases, interaction designs, and item page viewing histories.
- *Product development.* Big data analytics can provide details on the viability of new product ideas, choice-making throughout development, tracking of development activity, and ways to enhance products to better serve customers.
- *Price optimisation.* To extend benefits, retailers can select estimating models that show and utilise data from distinctive information sources.
- *Supply chain and channel investigation.* Prescient analytics models can offer assistance with proactive renewal, B2B provider systems, stock following, course optimisation and conveyance delay detailing.
- *Risk management.* For effective risk management techniques, big data analytics can find new dangers from data trends.
- *Improved decision-making.* Employing the knowledge that business users gain from relevant data allows organisations to make decisions more swiftly and efficiently.

3.11 USING DATA ANALYTICS TO COMBAT THE COVID-19 PANDEMIC

The COVID-19 outbreak, which accelerated at the end of 2019, was one of the most serious threats to the present health system. One of the most crucial applications was visualisation, which frequently educated the public on a variety of themes. To continuously update its database and give a more precise visual representation of the disease's severity, COVID-19 dashboards made use of access to publicly available data.

In analytics, these boards were used to identify hotspots and danger zones that could affect the transmission. Government agencies now use various lockdown procedures and security precautions for clinics, specialists, and other fundamental institutions as a result of comparative analyses.

The diagnosis of illnesses is another application. Reverse transcription polymerase chain reaction (RT-PCR), which is time-consuming and needs physical access to arrays, is currently the industry standard. To find out if the illness had affected the airways, a CT scan and chest X-ray were requested. A highly accurate deep CNN model was created using open-source image data. Patients with more critical diseases could receive priority care thanks to a quicker diagnosis, which would reduce the fatality rate.

Additionally, a number of investigations [10] have been made to identify drugs that can be utilised to treat the signs and symptoms of COVID-19. Numerous drugs have been selected for these researches, and the outcomes of those drugs have been investigated. Initiatives have also been taken to monitor the virus's transmission and spot potential outbreaks.

A COVID-19 application is used as an example to highlight the need of big data analytics in the healthcare industry. To forecast the fate of epidemics, X-rays, CT pictures, patient data, regional epidemic data, etc. are entered into a huge data system. Important conclusions from the investigation are displayed in Figure 3.6 and include contact tracking, diagnoses, immunisation recommendations, etc. Table 3.2 includes an overview of some of these activities, and Figure 3.6 displays COVID-19 data sources and analytics.

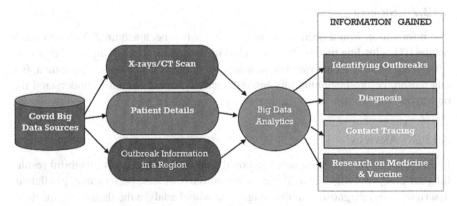

FIGURE 3.6 Big data analytics and sources from COVID-19.

TABLE 3.2
Analysis of data during the COVID-19 pandemic

Reference	Summary of Work	Topic of Concern
Rahmanti, Ningrum, Lazuardi, Yang, and Li (2021) [11]	Use of data mining and data analytics to the visualisation of epidemiology COVID-19 data. The idea of an original tool is put out; it is more adaptable and offers a clear grasp of patterns and trends.	Data visualisation for COVID-19
Wang et al. (2020) [12]	Classification of unlabelled data using a self-organising feature map (SOFM). According to this network, there were clear differences between radiographs of sick and healthy patients. The SOFM network was able to capture X-rays and extract features without a trained dataset.	Classification of chest X-rays using unsupervised learning
Calh, Sogancioglu, van Ginneken, van Leeuwen and Murphy (2021) [13]	Face mask detection is done via image classification. It uses the MobileNetV2 architecture to tell who is wearing a mask from who isn't, with a reported accuracy of 96.85%.	Detection of face masks

3.12 BIG DATA COMPONENTS

3.12.1 Ingestion

The act of gathering and getting ready the data is known as ingestion. You would prepare your data using the ETL (extract, transform, and load) procedure. You must choose your data sources in this step, decide whether to stream or collect data in batches, and prepare the data by organising, cleaning, and massaging it. In order to collect the data and optimise it, you must first complete the extract process.

3.12.2 Storage

The information would need to be stored once it had been acquired. You will carry out the ETL's loading process here, which is the last phase. Depending on your needs, either a data lake or a data warehouse would be where you would store your data. For this reason, before beginning any big data activity, it is essential to understand the objectives of your firm.

3.12.3 Analysis

In this stage of your big data process, you'd analyse the data to get insightful results for your company. Big data analytics come in four varieties: prescriptive, predictive, descriptive, and diagnostic. In this stage, you would analyse the data using machine learning and artificial intelligence techniques.

Fundamentals and Technicalities of Big Data and Analytics

3.12.4 CONSUMPTION

A big data procedure ends with this step. You must communicate your insights to others when you have analysed the data and discovered them. To effectively communicate your insights to a non-technical audience, such stakeholders and project managers, you would need to use data visualisation and data storytelling.

3.13 THE NECESSITY OF BIG DATA ANALYTICS AND TOOLS

Data from various data sources are processed and extracted using big data techniques. The value of big data is determined by more than just the amount of data available.

Figure 3.7 shows the predicted growth of the global data sphere from 33 Zettabytes in 2018 to 175 Zettabytes by 2025 according to Data Age 2025, a joint effort between Seagate and IDC [14]. What size is 175 ZB now? Accordingly, 1 ZB is equivalent to 1,000,000,000 GB (1 trillion GB). The stack of Blu-ray discs would reach the moon if 175 ZB were stored on them. According to B. S. Teh, senior vice-president of Seagate Technology, a top data and storage business, "the magnitude of increase of data is unprecedented and astonishing."

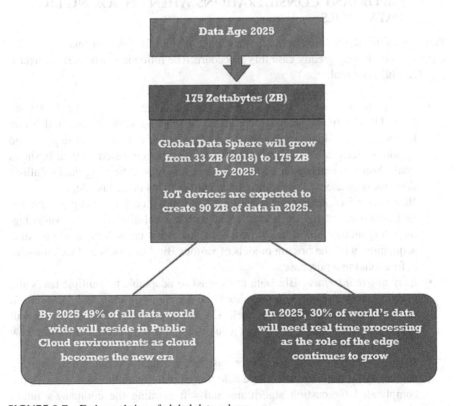

FIGURE 3.7 Estimated size of global data sphere.

The worth of something is determined by how it is used. The big data ecosystem is rapidly changing. Many analytical techniques are presently used to assist a wide range of business operations.

- To determine "what happened and why," users can use descriptive analysis. Such analysis includes scorecards and dashboards, as well as traditional survey and reporting options.
- Users can use predictive analytics to estimate the probability of a particular feature occurring. Examples include forecasting, fraud detection, preventive maintenance software, early warning systems and more.
- The user receives accurate (prescriptive) recommendations via prescriptive analytics. They provide a response to the query, "What should I do if 'x' occurs?"

Big data analytics can help forecast the future, boost corporate intelligence, and speed up decision making. Processing massive amounts of data in typical databases can be quite difficult. Big Data Tools consequently make it simple for you to manage your data.

3.14 IMPORTANT CONSIDERATIONS WHEN CHOOSING BIG DATA TOOLS

Your unique needs will determine the best big data tool for your business. Big Data integration tools may greatly ease this procedure. The following attributes are necessary for a big data tool:

- *Recognise the goals of your business:* A big data analytics platform, like any other IT investment, should be capable of meeting both present and future business needs. Begin by establishing a list of your company's core goals and important deliverables. Set quantitative analysis targets based on your business goals. You can reach your company objectives by selecting big data solutions that give data access and reporting capabilities. This is the last step.
- *Watch your budget:* Before selecting a Big Data Tool, you should completely understand all of the costs connected with the solution you are evaluating, including membership fees, growth costs, and other costs. You should become acquainted with the pricing models of various Big Data tools and technologies before making a purchase.
- *Easy-to-use interface:* Big Data tools must be adaptable to multiple users and usable. Dashboards and reports should be simple to develop and comprehend for non-technical personnel as well. Unattractive visuals on your panels will lower user adoption, especially if you're attempting to recruit and keep new employees.
- *Highly developed analytics:* To forecast future events and outcomes, your big data analytics platform should be able to find patterns in the data. Developing complicated forecasting algorithms and safeguarding the company's future

security necessitates contextual information in addition to simple mathematical calculations.
- *Smooth integrations:* When selecting a big data tool, consider if an integrated or stand-alone solution is better for your company. You have many possibilities with stand-alone solutions, but with integrated solutions, you get analytics from tools your staff is already familiar with. An analytics platform should be able to connect to both internal and external data sources.
- *Scalability and agility:* Cloud-hosted Big Data tools are designed to scale with your business. These compensation options might help firms gain a competitive advantage and stay afloat during periods of fast growth. Get faster access to information and use analytics to make better business decisions.
- *Strong protection:* In your big data environment, you might be working with sensitive data. As a result, you must evaluate the security of big data technologies to ensure that you have the appropriate controls in place to protect your data. Implement consistent security policies and procedures at all levels, processes, systems, and data to limit who has access to what information.

3.15 HOW DOES BIG DATA ANALYTICS FUNCTION?

Data analysts, data scientists, predictive modellers, statisticians, and other analysts collect, process, clean, and analyse increasing amounts of structured transactional data and other types of data not used by traditional business intelligence (BI) and analytics programs.

3.15.1 Four Steps in Big Data Analytics

The Big Data analytics process consists of four steps, which are summarised below.

Step 1: *Professionals gather information from a variety of sources.* Semi-structured and unstructured data are often mixed. Every organisation uses different data streams, such as Internet click-streams; mobile apps; social media posts; Web server logs; cloud services; customer emails and review responses; cell phone records; and appliance data collected from IoT-connected sensors.

Step 2: *Data processing and preparation.* After collecting and storing data from a data lake or warehouse, data experts must properly segment, organise, and structure the data for analytical questions. Data is carefully prepared and processed to achieve better performance from analytical queries.

Step 3: *Cleaning is done to enhance data quality.* Data experts clean the data using scripting tools or software for data quality improvement. They sort and clean the data and look for duplicates or formatting errors.

Step 4: Utilising analytics software, the information is gathered, edited, and cleansed. There are tools for:

- Searching for patterns and links in large data sets is known as data mining.
- Predictive analytics is the process of developing models to forecast customer behaviour as well as other upcoming events, scenarios, and trends.

- Machine learning, which examines large data sets using a variety of techniques.
- A more sophisticated branch of machine learning is called deep learning.
- Software for statistical analysis and text mining
- Artificial Intelligence (AI)
- Popular business intelligence software
- Tools for data visualisation

3.16 IMPORTANT TECHNOLOGY AND TOOLS FOR BIG DATA ANALYTICS

Big data analytics processes are supported by a wide range of tools and technologies. The technologies and tools listed below are frequently used in big data analysis processes.

- *Hadoop* could be a free and open source system for organising and storing enormous data. It is capable of storing massive amounts of data both, structured and unstructured.
- *Predictive analytics technology and software* can analyse vast amounts of complex data and forecast the outcomes of events using statistical and machine learning methods. For fraud detection, marketing, risk assessment, and operational purposes, businesses utilise predictive analytics solutions.
- *Tools for stream analytics*, which can be saved in various designs or stages and used to filter, sum, and analyse mass data.
- *Distributed storage of data*, typically on a non-relational database, which is replicated. Providing low-latency access or protecting against independent node failures, lost or damaged huge data, are some examples of possible uses for this.
- *NoSQL databases* are effective while handling huge distributed data volumes and non-relational data management systems. They work best with unstructured and raw data because they don't need a set format.
- A *data lake* can be a huge capacity space where crude information is kept in its normal shape until it is required. Data lakes utilise a level design.
- *Data warehouse* is a depository of mass data collected from different source. Data warehouses often utilise predetermined schemas to store data.
- Tools for mining massive amounts of big data, both organised and unstructured, known as *knowledge extraction data mining* tools.
- *In-memory data infrastructure* spreads out big volumes of data over system memory resources. This makes it possible to obtain and interpret data with little delay.
- *Data virtualisation* makes it possible to access data without facing any technical limitations.
- *Data integration tools* make it possible to simplify massive data across a variety of platforms, such as Apache, Hadoop, Amazon EMR and MongoDB.
- *Data quality tools* purge and augment huge data sets.

/ Fundamentals and Technicalities of Big Data and Analytics

- *Tool for pre-processing data* so that it is ready for additional analysis unstructured data is cleaned, and data is prepared.
- *Spark*: for processing batch and stream data, the open source cluster computing framework Spark is employed.

Most early big data systems were placed locally, especially in significant businesses that collected, organised, and analysed enormous volumes of data. However, setting up and managing Hadoop clusters on the cloud has become simpler thanks to cloud platform providers like Amazon Web Services (AWS), Google, and Microsoft. AWS, Google, and Microsoft Azure all enable Hadoop deployment, as do other Hadoop service providers like Cloudera.

With usage-based pricing that does not require continuous software licences, users can now create cloud-based clusters, run them for however long they are required to, and then take them offline.

Advanced analytics, such as big data analytics, differ noticeably from conventional business intelligence (BI) in a number of key ways.

3.17 BIG DATA TOOLS IN HEALTHCARE

Before being made available to the scientific community, healthcare data must be saved in an easy-to-access and understandable file format for effective analysis. Another vital aspect of health information is the application of advanced computing strategies, strategies, and technology in clinical setup. Apache Hadoop, MongoDB, Lumify, Scene, Kaggle, Hive, R, Oozie, Knime and Data wrapper are the most popular open source big data tools in healthcare analytics. We've discussed a few devices in terms of their importance in a large data framework [15].

- A healthy analytics system can be built with the help of Hadoop. But, as mentioned earlier, this is only a batch system. Due to the patient's heart rate is detected in milliseconds, it cannot fully utilise in real-time emergencies such as ECG readings [15].
- In multi-pass analytics, Apache Spark can be 100 times faster than Hadoop due to in-memory data processing. This is possible because robust distributed datasets are provided. The Spark platform is used in healthcare for big data analytics. It makes use of its streaming capability to execute better analysis without even additional supports [16].
- The Apache Flink platform is perfect for event-driven applications. Additionally, the traditional reactive to proactive shift in health analytics is required. For applications requiring real-time health monitoring, a streaming platform is a great choice [17].

When choosing whether to utilise a big data platform in healthcare arrangement, real-time necessities, information volume, speed, adaptability, and execution are being considered. For a few healthcare administrations, such as EMR records, where real-time data isn't required, a non-streaming stage such as Hadoop or MapReduce can be used. Adaptability isn't an issue, as a few applications such as ECG investigation require real-time reaction, requiring the use of live gushing. A few proposal applications, such as symptomatic suggestion bolster, require a platform that can scale and acknowledge gigantic sums of information; in this case, flat scaling frameworks like Spark are exceptionally valuable, but vertical frameworks like CUDA or high-performance Computing are wasteful.

Fault tolerance is another issue to consider. This speaks to the platform's resilience to failure. Vertical scaling stages have a single point of malfunction, whereas horizontal scaling frameworks, such as Hadoop and Spark, distribute work across multiple clusters, albeit not equally.

Health analytics administrations are sold by IBM Organization. Clinics, suppliers and analysts can share and analyse health information utilising AI's Watson Health platform.

3.18 BENEFITS OF BIG DATA ANALYTICS

Here are some of the benefits of big data analytics:

- Rapidly analyse colossal amounts of information from diverse sources in several formats and types.
- Quickly make more informed vital planning conclusions that can upgrade and progress supply chain, operations and other making vital decisions.
- Savings as a result of new and enhanced business procedures.
- Better thoughtful of client requirements, behaviour and emotions, which can lead to more accurate market observation and product expansion data.
- Advanced risk management solutions that are more educated and based on huge data sample sizes.

3.19 TECHNOLOGY FOR STORING BIG DATA

This kind of big data technology consists of storage, retrieval, and management infrastructure. Data is set up so that various programmes can easily access, use, and process it. Top big data tools for this kind of data work include the following.

3.19.1 HADOOP TECHNOLOGIES

The MapReduce programming model is a framework included in the Hadoop technology stack for distributed storage and massive data processing. One benefit of using this Apache big data stack is its speedy management of dispersed data (storage and processing) at affordable prices. Big data solutions like Hadoop are scalable, fault-tolerant, and incredibly adaptable. Hadoop has drawbacks such as limited support for massive data files, batch processing only, and inadequate security. The Hadoop technology stack can be replaced by big data technologies and spark tools.

Fundamentals and Technicalities of Big Data and Analytics

3.19.2 MongoDB

One of the big data database technologies is MongoDB, a NoSQL programme that works with JSON-like documents. It offers a different schema from relational databases. This makes it possible to manage a variety of data that are present throughout distributed architectures in significant quantities. MongoDB's key benefits are flexibility and scalability. This is because using replica sets with this big data database is simple. MongoDB, on the other side, is poor in that it moves slowly and stores more data.

3.19.3 Rainstor

This database management system software manages huge data for enterprises. As it goes through and stores enormous amounts of data for reference, it can remove duplicate files. The most recent version of this programme can manage large data volumes with high ingest rates. It also supports cloud storage and has multi-tenancy features. Large data sets can be shrunk via Rainstor for cloud storage. A terabyte can be condensed to 25 GB. Reduced costs are one of Rainstor's additional benefits.

3.20 THE STORAGE OF TOMORROW

3.20.1 Hard Disk Drives

According to Seagate's CFO, replacing the hard disc will take another 15–20 years. It is now one of the oldest computing technologies. The Advanced Storage Technology Consortium has proposed a technology roadmap that predicts that by 2025, HDDs would have a capacity of 100 terabytes (TB), made possible by new writing techniques such helium-filled casings, perpendicular magnetic recording, and shingled magnetic recording.

3.20.2 Helium Drives

On the outside, helium drives resemble HDDs exactly. The most important factor is what's inside. Helium drives store data on platters that are physically identical to those used by HDDs, but helium, not air, and is pumped into the enclosed enclosure. Helium has a density that is six times lower than that of air, hence spinning the discs requires much less force due to the reduced resistance. The same-shaped layer houses numerous stations, while the temperature remains cooler due to the cooler structure. Helium drives provide new levels of performance through trustworthy technology, but they do not represent a fundamental shift in data storage. They are also just going to get more economical.

3.20.3 DNA Storage

Nucleic acid strands have long been read, put together, and even synthesised. Scientists have recently been able to chemically create a sequence of nucleotides that represent data by translating binary information into DNA bases (A, G, T, and C).

Although writing is a time-consuming and costly procedure, DNA strands offer a very dense and durable method of storage. According to the researchers, if properly stored in a cold, dark environment, DNA may safely store information and be ready for error-free recovery for up to a million years. Today's hard drives would eventually have trouble operating. Due to the much specialised technology needed to convert data into a format that can be read by conventional computers, DNA storage may never be used in residential buildings. Furthermore, encoding 83 KB of data now costs roughly $2,000. However, it has a lot of promise for usage in both science and industry.

3.20.4 Holographic Storage

In contrast to magnetic and disc-based media, which store individual bits in two-dimensional physical space, holographic storage makes use of photosensitive optical material to simultaneously store multiple bits of data by using light from various angles.

In contrast to a flat surface, data can now be stored in a three-dimensional volume. Similar data is kept on several layers on physical media like DVDs, but the laser can only read in one direction at once.

3.21 STRATEGIES FOR ANALYSING BIG DATA

This section addresses the following major categories of data analysis techniques:

- Quantitative analysis
- Qualitative analysis
- Data mining
- Statistical analysis
- Machine learning
- Semantic analysis
- Visual analysis

3.21.1 Quantitative Analysis

The goal of quantitative analysis is to detect and quantify patterns and relationships in data. This statistical method necessitates a large number of material observations. The results of a quantitative analysis are quantitative in nature. The results of quantitative analyses may be compared numerically because they are absolute in nature. A quantitative analysis of ice cream sales, for example, might discover that a 5 degree increase in temperature improves sales by 15%.

3.21.2 Qualitative Analysis

A data analysis method known as qualitative analysis relies on verbally defining distinct data properties. Additionally, they cannot be numerically quantified or compared. A review of ice cream sales, for instance, might show that June's sales were higher than those of May. The findings in the analysis give no numerical difference, just stating that the numbers were "not as high as." The result of a qualitative analysis is a verbal description of the relationship.

3.21.3 Data Mining

A specific type of data analysis that focuses on huge databases is called data mining, commonly referred to as data discovery. In the context of big data analysis, data mining is frequently used to describe automated software approaches that analyse massive data sets for patterns and trends. It primarily refers to extracting hidden or undiscovered patterns from data with the purpose of discovering undiscovered patterns. Analytics and business intelligence that uses predictions are based on data mining (BI).

3.21.4 Statistical Analysis

In statistical analysis, data is analysed using statistical techniques based on mathematical formulas. Though it can also be qualitative, statistical analysis is most frequently quantitative. This sort of analysis is frequently used to summarise data and generate statistics like mean, median, and mode. It can also be used to infer patterns and relationships in a data set by employing regression and correlation.

3.21.4.1 Types of Statistical Analysis
- A/B testing
- Correlation
- Regression

3.21.4.1.1 A/B Testing

Split or cluster testing, also known as A/B testing, compares two versions of an item to see which one is superior based on a predetermined criterion. Numerous items might make up the element. An offer for a good or service, like discounts on electronics, or content, like a Web page, are two examples. The treatment refers to the modified version of the element, whereas the control refers to the element as it is currently. Concurrent experimentation is conducted on both versions. To establish which version is more successful, the observations are kept.

3.21.4.1.2 Correlation

The analysis method of correlation is used to ascertain whether two variables are connected to one another. The following stage is to establish their relationship if it is discovered that they are related. For instance, Variable A's value rises every time Variable B's value rises. We may be interested in studying how much variable B grows relative to the increase in variable A to see how closely variables A and B are related.

For example, managers think that ice cream shops should stock more ice cream on hot days, but they are not sure how much more. To find out if there is a relationship between temperature and ice cream sales, analysts first use a correlation between the amount of ice cream sold and the observed temperature readings.

A correlation of +0.75 indicates a significant association between the two. This correlation suggests that ice cream sales grow with rising temperatures.

3.21.4.1.3 Regression

Regression analysis investigates the relationships between a dataset's dependent and independent variables. The nature of the relationship between the independent variable of temperature and the dependent variable of crop yield can be determined using regression.

The analysts use regression, for example, feeding in temperature readings to predict how much additional stock each ice cream shop needs. These numbers are based on a dependent variable, the quantity of ice creams sold, and an independent variable, the weather forecast.

To start with, one can utilise correlation to see if there is a relationship in massive data. Regression can be used to investigate the relationship and predict the values of the dependent variable based on the known values of the independent variable.

3.21.5 Machine Learning

Humans can perceive links and patterns in data. Unfortunately, we cannot evaluate large amounts of data quickly. Machines, on the other hand, can quickly assimilate massive amounts of data if they are trained to do. If people' experience and machine speed can be coupled, robots will be able to process massive amounts of data without the assistance of humans. This is the fundamental idea of machine learning.

Various kinds of machine learning methods:

- Classification (supervised ML)
- Clustering (unsupervised ML)
- Outlier detection
- Filtering

Data is categorised using the supervised learning technique of classification into pertinent, previously discovered categories. Healthcare industries can benefit from classification [18, 19].

By grouping data into several categories so that the data in each category has characteristics in common, clustering is an unsupervised learning technique. There is no prerequisite for category knowledge. The segmentation of brain tissues in magnetic resonance imaging can also be done via clustering [20–23].

Finding data within a dataset that differs considerably from or is inconsistent with other data is a technique known as outlier detection. Anomalies and irregularities in healthcare are identified using this machine learning technique.

Finding pertinent items automatically from a pool of items is a process known as filtering.

Fundamentals and Technicalities of Big Data and Analytics

3.21.6 Semantic Analysis

A whole sentence may still have the same meaning even if it is organised differently than a segment of text or voice, which can have several meanings depending on the context. Robots need to understand text and speech data just like humans do to extract useful information. The process of collecting meaningful information from speech and text data is known as semantic analysis.

There are many kinds of semantic analysis:

- Natural language processing (NLP)
- Text analytics
- Sentiment analysis

3.21.7 Visual Analysis

Data is graphically presented as part of visual analysis to aid or enhance visual perception. Visual analysis functions as a Big Data perception tool based on the notion that images are easier to interpret and draw conclusions from than text.

The purpose is to better grasp the content being examined by using graphical representations. It is especially useful for detecting and highlighting hidden patterns, connections, and anomalies. Visual analysis and exploratory data analysis are inextricably linked.

There are many forms of visual analysis:

- Heat maps
- Time series plots
- Network graphs
- Spatial data mapping

3.22 BIG DATA TECHNOLOGY TYPES

Big Data technologies aim to assist users in storing, managing, integrating, processing, and finding answers for their problems, as was previously discussed. Operational and analytical are two broad divisions that can be used to categorise the numerous big data technologies and methodologies.

3.22.1 Operational

Many big data engineers, IT specialists, and networking professionals work together on this side of big data technologies to handle and store enormous amounts of data.

These are the technologies that are in charge of producing huge data and effectively storing it but not of offering any solutions. These data may come from social media platforms, online stores, hospitality-related businesses like ticketing data, or internal sources within the company.

The management and storage of this data is the responsibility of the organisations. As a result, big data technology grows organically from an organisation's day-to-day activities and supports its analytical skills.

3.22.2 ANALYTICAL

Data scientists and analysts are useful in this situation. They make use of the Big Data technologies that aid in the analysis of massive amounts of data to identify business solutions. Here, typical analytics techniques are put to use, such as stock marketing forecasts, weather predictions, early disease detection for insurance businesses, etc.

3.23 LEADING TECHNOLOGIES AND TECHNIQUES FOR BIG DATA

Big data tools are typically grouped based on how useful they are. As indicated in Figure 3.8, big data technologies and approaches can be broadly classified into four primary categories: storage, analytics, mining, and visualisation.

3.23.1 DATA STORAGE TOOLS

3.23.1.1 Hadoop

Hadoop, a prominent big data solution, is used to process data in a clustered mode, or when data is divided into smaller chunks for user consumption. It is essentially a Big Data management system that employs an odd distribution scheme. Hadoop Common, YARN (Yet Another Resource Negotiator), MapReduce, and HDFS (Hadoop Distributed File System) are significant parts of the HADOOP ecosystem.

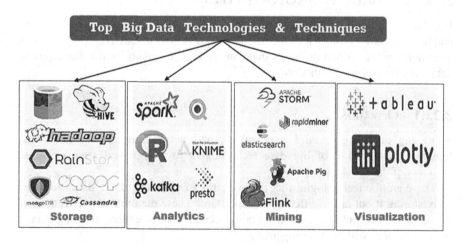

FIGURE 3.8 Big data technologies and methodologies fall into four broad areas.

So, there are three sections:

- HDFS, the Hadoop Distributed File System, is the storage layer.
- Hadoop's map-reduce framework is used for data processing.
- Resource management for Hadoop is done through YARN.

Pros: Java-based, strong parallel processing capability, simple installation superior availability, dependable data protection.

Cons: need advanced training, has a high processing power requirement, elaborate integrations, no capability for real-time processing, no memory-based calculations.

3.23.1.2 HIVE

HIVE is a significant tool in the field of large data tools because to its ability to efficiently extract, read, and write data. It employs the same query-based language, Hive Query Language (HQL), supports all SQL data types, and includes drivers (JDBC drivers) and a command line. It also employs the same SQL technique and interface (HIVE Command-Line).

3.23.1.3 MongoDB

In terms of storage, this is yet another instrument crucial for large data. As a NoSQL-based database, MongoDB differs from traditional RDBMS databases in some ways. Large volumes of data can be stored easily because it doesn't employ the conventional schema and data structure. MongoDB is renowned for its efficiency and adaptability with a variety of distributed systems.

Pros: Strong load balancing skills, the server less option, very user-friendly.

Cons: More slowly paced processing, multifaceted integrations, customer service is too slow.

3.23.1.4 Apache Sqoop

Using this tool, huge data may be transferred from Apache Hadoop to structured data storage like MYSQL and Oracle and vice versa. It offers connectors for each of the main RDBMS.

3.23.1.5 RainStor

Database administration software called RainStor was created by the firm named as the software itself. It offers an enterprise online data archiving solution that utilises HDFS natively and runs on top of Hadoop. It employs a process known as deduplication techniques to store vast volumes of data.

3.23.1.6 Data Lakes

A data lake is a centralised data warehouse where all sorts of data, including raw data, are stored. As there is no need to convert the data into a structured format before storing it, the data gathering process is simplified, and many big data-based technologies can be employed to do analysis.

3.23.1.7 Cassandra

It is a distinct instrument for storing large amounts of data. It's a NoSQL database that can manage data from various clusters. Because of its scalability, query-based language functionality, MapReduce interface, and distributed technique, it is often the most popular choice for NoSQL databases.

- By giving users lower latency, support for replicating across various data centres.
- Automatic data replication across numerous nodes provides fault tolerance.
- It's one of the top big data solutions and works best for applications that simply cannot afford to lose data, even when an entire data centre is unavailable.
- Third-party services are also offered by Cassandra, who also offers support contracts.

3.23.2 BIG DATA TOOLS WITH DATA ANALYTICS

3.23.2.1 Apache Spark

Spark is a critical component of Big Data, allowing users to execute operations such as batch processing, interactive or iterative processing, visualisation, manipulation, and so on. Because it uses RAM, it is substantially faster than many previous big data solutions. Its competitor Hadoop is frequently used for structured and batch processing, whereas Spark is frequently utilised for real-time data, allowing businesses to use both tools concurrently.

It includes powerful Java, Python, Scala, and R APIs. Furthermore, Spark provides a large range of sophisticated tools such as Spark SQL for structured data processing, MLlib for machine learning, GraphX for processing graph datasets, and Spark Streaming. It also has 80 high-level operators for quickly processing queries.

Pros: Open-source sophisticated drivers that are more adaptive and versatile than Hadoop real-time and batch processing, as well as in-memory calculations, are supported.

Cons: Necessary advanced training, the value of documentation varies, necessary additional security measures.

3.23.2.2 R-language

The programming language R is frequently referred to as a language created by statisticians for statisticians. It aids scientists and data analysts in running statistical analyses and building statistical models. But models based on machine learning and deep learning can also be built using R. Due to its ability to be integrated with big data-based technologies, R made this list.

3.23.2.3 QlikView

QlikView, a very potent business intelligence (BI) solution, aids in producing quick and in-depth insights from massive data. It includes an easy-to-use interface that enables users to perform unconstrained data analyses by just clicking on data points. Associative data modelling is used to aid in determining the association between features in one dataset or other datasets.

3.23.2.4 Qlik Sense

The drag-and-drop user interface of Qlik Sense, like that of QlikView, makes it simple for users to quickly build reports with narrative structure.

3.23.2.5 Hunk

Hunk is a large data tool for exploring, analysing, and visualising Hadoop data. It allows for drag-and-drop analysis, a flexible developer environment, client dashboards, integrated analysis, and rapid deployment. It analyses data using the Splunk Search Processing Language.

3.23.2.6 Platfora

It is a subscription-based big data platform that supports big data analysis. It is a user-friendly tool for early pattern recognition and raw data processing.

3.23.2.7 Kafka

Similar to an enterprise messaging system, Kafka is a platform for stream processing. It handles a lot of real-time data sources and distributes them. It is utilised for data processing, real-time data distribution, etc.

3.23.2.8 Presto

Big data analytics frequently employ this technology. It employs the Distributed SQL Query engine, which has been designed specifically for use with Interactive Analytics Queries. Various data sources, including Hive, Cassandra, MYSQL, etc., can be used with Presto. It facilitates the execution of pipelines, the development of user-defined functions, and elementary code debugging. Last but not least, the largest benefit is that it scales well with high data velocity, which is why businesses like Facebook has developed Presto-based apps for their data analytics requirements.

3.23.2.9 KNIME

This Java-based big data application enables users to employ complex data mining techniques, data extraction with SQL queries, predictive analytics, and other features in workflow and data analysis.

Additionally, it may leverage MLlib integration to connect to popular Hadoop distributions and use machine learning methods.

Uses of KNIME

- Don't create code blocks. Instead, you need to drag-and-drop connection points between tasks.
- Programming languages are supported by this data analysis tool.
- In reality, these types of analysis tools can be expanded to run R, Python, Text Mining, and Chemistry data.

KNIME's limitations: Inadequate data visualisation.

3.23.2.10 Splunk

This big data tool offers instant data insights. The user can connect to tools like Tableau and various databases like Oracle, MYSQL, etc. and access Hadoop clusters through virtual indexes. By helping the user to index, collect and compare such data, it facilitates the processing of real-time streaming data. Additionally, users can quickly gain insights by creating reports, charts, dashboards, etc.

3.23.2.11 Mahout

Mahout allows machine learning to be applied to massive data and performs ML-based operations such as segmentation, classification, collaborative filtering, and so on.

3.24 BIG DATA TOOLS EMPLOYING DATA MINING

3.24.1 MapReduce

MapReduce can manage the volume component of Big Data because it uses parallel and distributed algorithms to execute reasoning on enormous data sets. As a result, MapReduce is required to turn otherwise incomprehensible data into a reasonable structure. It combines the terms "Map" and "Reduce," the word "MapReduce" is a portmanteau. Reduce is essential for summarising and aggregating data whereas Map is in charge of data sorting and filtering.

3.24.2 Apache PIG

Pig Latin, a query-based language created by Yahoo and used for structuring, processing, and analysing massive data, is akin to SQL. It offers programming simplicity by enabling users to design their own unique functions and converting them behind the scenes into the MapReduce programme.

3.24.3 RapidMiner

ETL, data mining, predictive modelling, and machine learning are just a few of the many tasks it may carry out. Because it supports different languages, assists

Fundamentals and Technicalities of Big Data and Analytics

in resolving issues with business analytics, and has an easy-to-use user interface, RapidMiner is a beneficial tool. One of its main benefits is that it is open-source, which is nevertheless regarded as secure in most cases while being open-sourced. *RapidMiner's drawbacks*:

- Regarding the number of rows, RapidMiner is subject to size restrictions.
- In comparison to ODM and SAS, RapidMiner requires larger hardware resources.

3.24.4 Apache Storm

Storm is an open source scalable distributed real-time computing system. It aids in handling the processing of unlimited streams of data because it is based on Java and Clojure.

- It is one of the most powerful technologies on the market, processing one million 100-byte messages per second per node.
- Big data techniques and technology that leverage parallel processing across numerous sets of devices are included.
- If a node fails, it will restart automatically. The worker will start over on a different node.
- Storm promises to process each data unit at least once or exactly once.
- The simplest tool for big data analysis once implemented is Storm.

3.24.5 Flink

To handle both finite and unbounded data streams, Apache Flink was created. Although processing of bounded data is similar to batch processing, it has a distinct beginning and finish. Flink is thus a highly scalable distributed processing engine. Both applications for data analytics and pipelines for data can use Flink.

- It provides trustworthy results even when data arrives out of order or late; it is stateful, error tolerant, and capable of recovering from faults.
- It is a big data analytics program that operates on thousands of nodes and can provide high-volume performance.
- It has favourable throughput and latency properties.
- It enables customizable windowing for data-driven windows based on time, count, or sessions.
- It supports a variety of third-party system connectors for data sources and sinks.

3.24.6 Elastic Search

It is a prominent Java-based search engine used by numerous businesses (e.g., Accenture, Stack Overflow, Netflix, etc.). It includes a full-text search engine powered by Lucene, an HTTP web interface, and schema-free JSON files.

3.25 TOOLS FOR BIG DATA WITH DATA VISUALISATION

3.25.1 Tableau

Tableau, a sophisticated data visualisation tool, can now interact with spreadsheets, big data platforms, the cloud, relational databases, and other systems, giving users rapid access to unstructured data. Because it is a safe, proprietary solution that also enables for real-time dashboard sharing, this product is gaining popularity.

Pros: Searches with no code and visualisation, simple setup, instantaneous cooperation, streamlined integrations.

Cons: More costly than certain tools, difficulties with customer service.

3.25.2 Plotly

Using the Plotly library, users may build interactive dashboards. For every popular language, including Python, R, MATLAB, and Julia, it offers API libraries. One tool that makes it simple to create interactive graphs in Python is Plotly Dash.

3.26 LATEST BIG DATA TECHNOLOGIES AND TOOLS

Numerous cutting-edge big data technologies will be in high demand. Since big data technologies are always evolving, it is crucial for those interested in a career in data science to understand them and have a working knowledge of their fundamentals.

3.26.1 Docker

Users may create, test, deploy, and operate their apps using Docker. It makes use of the idea of containers, a system for splitting software into uniform components. It is advantageous for the user to package his application so that all of its components, including system tools and dependent libraries, are located in a single location. Docker aids in standardising application functionality, lowering expenses, and improving overall deployment dependability.

3.26.2 Tensor Flow

AI is growing more popular in the Big Data field, and Tensor Flow, a self-contained ecosystem of resources, modules, and tools, is one of the front-runners. Tensor Flow can be used to create machine learning and deep learning models for use with large amounts of data.

3.26.3 Apache Beam

Parallel data processing pipelines are made using it. Processing huge amounts of data is facilitated by this. In order to define the pipeline, the user must create a programme, which can be written in Java, Python, Go, etc.

3.26.4 KUBERNETES

By automating the deployment and scaling of containerised apps across host clusters, this Big Data tool aids the user. Kubernetes makes it simple to monitor containerised apps deployed in the cloud.

3.26.5 BLOCKCHAIN

By producing encrypted data blocks and linking them together, big data technology makes it possible to interact with digital currencies like bitcoin in a very secure manner. Big data has a lot of potential uses for blockchain, so many that the banking, financial services, and insurance (BFSI) industry is prepared to take use of them.

3.26.6 AIRFLOW

A scheduling and pipeline tool is Apache Airflow. It aids in the planning and administration of intricate data pipelines originating from numerous sources. These workflows are represented as Directed Acyclic Graphs (DAG) in this tool. Airflow aids with the creation and management of data pipelines, increasing the efficacy and accuracy of ML models.

3.27 NEW BIG DATA TOOLS IN 2022

3.27.1 ZOHO ANALYTICS

Zoho Analytics is a low-cost and user-friendly big data analytics tool for small enterprises. Its user interface is simple to use, making it simple to design comprehensive dashboards and rapidly locate the most crucial information.

3.27.2 XPLENTY

Xplenty, a cloud-based data integration platform, simplifies data from a variety of structured, unstructured, and semi-structured sources. It is a low-code ETL platform that enriches, transforms, and cleans each dataset before transporting it to the data warehouse. It's frequently used in tandem with other tools like Tableau.

3.27.3 ATLAS.TI

Atlas.ti is software that allows you to conduct all of your research in one spot. You may use this big data analyser to connect to all available platforms. It can be utilised in academic, marketing, and user experience research for mixed methodologies and qualitative data analysis.

3.27.4 HPCC

HPCC, a big data tool developed by LexisNexis Risk Solution, was built. It offers services via a single platform, architecture, and programming language.

- One of the most capable big data tools, it performs big data with substantially less code.
- It is a huge data processing tool with high availability and redundancy.
- Both simple and extensive data processing can be done with it on a Thor cluster.
- Development, testing, and debugging are made simpler by graphic IDEs.
- It automatically turns ECL code into efficient C++ for parallel processing, and it may also be expanded using C++ libraries.

3.27.5 STATS IQ

An intuitive statistical tool is Stats iQ from Qualtrics. Big data analysts constructed it for them. Automatic statistical test selection is made by its contemporary interface.

- It is a large data tool capable of rapidly exploring any data.
- With Statwing, you can quickly make charts, discover relationships, and tidy up data.
- It enables the creation of bar charts, heat maps, scatterplots, and histograms that can be exported to PowerPoint or Excel.
- Analysts who are not familiar with statistical analysis might use it to translate results into plain English.

3.27.6 CouchDB

CouchDB allows for web access and JavaScript-based querying. It saves data in JSON documents. This provides safe storage and distributed scalability. It gives access to data by keeping a log of each reproduction.

- Unlike other databases, CouchDB is a single-node database.
- One approach of processing enormous amounts of data allows for the use of a single logical database server on an infinite number of servers.
- JSON data format and the widely used HTTP protocol are both utilised.
- Database replication across several server instances is simple.
- Simple interface for document retrieval, insertion, changes, and deletion.
- Language translation is possible for the JSON-based document format.

3.27.7 Pentaho

Pentaho offers tools for extracting, preparing, and blending big data. It offers visuals and data that transform how any business is run. Big data can be transformed into big insights using this technique.

Fundamentals and Technicalities of Big Data and Analytics 89

- To effectively visualise data, data must be accessed and integrated.
- It is a big data program that enables companies to collect and transmit enormous amounts of data at the source for correct analysis.
- It switches processes effortlessly or combines them for cluster execution for maximum computing power.
- Analytical tools, such as charts, visualisations, and reporting, make it simple to check data.
- It provides special features to support a broad range of big data sources.

3.27.8 Cloudera

The most quick, simple, and most secure big data platform is called Cloudera. It enables anyone to access all data from any environment via a single scalable platform.

- It is a high-performing big data analytics software.
- It includes a multi-cloud option
- Cloudera Enterprise may be deployed and managed on AWS, Azure, and Google Cloud Platform.
- It can be used to create and remove clusters, and spend money only when necessary.
- It aids in creating and educating data models.
- It provides immediate insights for detection and monitoring.

3.27.9 Openrefine

An effective large data tool is Openrefine. With the aid of cleaning and format conversion, this big data analytics tool makes it possible to work with unorganised data. The addition of web services and outside data is also possible.

- It can be used to combine and expand the dataset using different online services.
- It can import data in multiple formats.
- Data sets can be searched in seconds.
- Data sets can be linked instantly together.
- To automatically find themes in text fields, use named-entity extraction.
- Sophisticated data operations can be utlised by Improve Expression Language.

3.27.10 Google Fusion Tables

We have a more stylish, more expansive version of Google Spreadsheets when it comes to data tools. It is a fantastic tool for data analysis, mapping, and large-scale dataset display. Another tool for business analytics is Google Fusion Tables. The greatest Big Data analytics tools include this one as well.

Applications of Google Fusion Tables:

- Data from larger tables can be seen online.
- Over a million rows of data can be filtered and summarised.
- Tables can be combined with other online information.
- To create a single visualisation with sets of data, combine two or three tables. A map may be made in a few minutes!

Limitations of Google Fusion Tables:

- The query results or maps only contain the first 100,000 rows of data from a table.
- 1 MB is the maximum amount of data that can be supplied in one API call.

3.27.11 KAGGLE

The biggest big data community on the planet is Kaggle. By posting their data and statistics on the Kaggle, organisations and researchers benefit. Data analysis can be done there most effectively.

- It is the top location for finding and easily analysing open data.
- Open datasets can be found using the search bar.
- You can get involved in the open data movement and network with other data enthusiasts.

3.28 THE HEALTHCARE SECTOR UNDERGOES VARIOUS PHASES

This section examines the five stages of Big Data analytics and their importance in increasing health applications and research. The large amount of structured, unstructured, and semi-structured data created by today's healthcare systems or organisations is collected, processed, analysed, reviewed, and managed utilising specialised analytical tools and techniques.

The following is a summary of the major parts of large health data analytics, from data mining to the knowledge discovery process:

Phase 1: Data gathering, compiling, and storing

The first phase aims to collect various health data from billions of sources (i.e., internal and external sources). As described in the previous section, the information we collect can come in many different forms. Once transmitted, it is either stored in databases or a data warehouse, or delivered to a system for analysis. Healthcare processing is complex due to a lack of data standards, protocols and scalability, as well as privacy concerns.

Cleaning up data is a crucial issue. If the information that has been stored is unusable, the processing error may increase as it goes through the complete data analysis step.

Fundamentals and Technicalities of Big Data and Analytics

Phase 2: Cleansing, eliminating, and classifying data
Specifically, this second stage is utilised to extract and store medical information on a single database. Inaccurate health-related records are found and eliminated using the data cleansing procedure. The information gathered from sensors, doctor's prescriptions, medical picture data, and social networking data is frequently not in an inaccurate format because the data needs to be in an organised manner to do the proper analysis. At this point, subtracting and adding missing data is a constant challenge. For example, the generated data may comprise medical pictures (e.g., MRI, CT, PET/CT, and ultrasound), which are frequently difficult to filter based on their structure. This data must be classified into three types for useful analysis: structured, semi-structured, and unstructured data.

Phase 3: Integrating, acquiring, and representing data
This stage aggregates the accumulated large and diverse amount of medical data so that it may be used efficiently for data analysis. The primary purpose is to gather detailed information on individual patient records based on criteria such as creation date, similarity to other records, critical condition, patient name, history of previous readings, and so on. Hospitals, data scientists, researchers, and local, state, regional, and national health institutions will eventually obtain aggregated data.

Because combining dynamic medical data with existing static data in real time is a difficult task. Healthcare workers need accurate and current patient information in order to diagnose and treat diseases.

Phase 4: Processing queries and modelling data
The complex medical data is transformed into a simple to grasp format utilising graphs, text, and symbols during the data modelling step. It is primarily used to observe the same health data and verify the identification of all processes, entities, linkages, and data flows.

The purpose of data analysis is to extract relevant information from health datasets using various analytical approaches and methodologies such as data mining algorithms.

Querying the valuable data comes after the medical data has been combined and analysed. A method of answering user-level requests is query processing.

Phase 5: Comprehension, dissemination, and evaluation of data
Data interpretation, data distribution, and feedback comprise the big data analytics phase's final stages. After completing all of the aforementioned data processing procedures, data interpretation is crucial. The findings of the analysis of the healthcare data should be quite straightforward. If this is unclear, patients and other healthcare professionals cannot understand the results of the data analyst, decision maker, or even computer systems.

The data transfer step helps create a health report based on the previous data model. This model will help clinicians administer the appropriate care to stop any more issues.

In order to improve the standard of patient care, decision-makers and patients will provide suggestions throughout the final phase.

3.29 A CASE STUDY USING BIG DATA IN HEALTHCARE

The blood glucose level differs in every human being causing a metabolic disorder termed as diabetes mellitus.

It may occur due to insufficient insulin formation (type-1 diabetes) or incapability to develop insulin (type-2 diabetes) in the body. Nowadays, diabetes is widespread among the people of any age. It has become essential to detect the disease early on for the betterment of life. In recent healthcare systems, the dealing with physical files and accessing them for examination have become cumbersome. For this reason, healthcare industry is looking for data analytics to analyse these kinds of data. Hence, the healthcare sector is seeking effective IT tools for providing better treatment experience to the patient.

3.29.1 Objective

The purpose of this study is to assess the database of diabetic patients by a blend of hierarchical decision attention network, association rules (AR), and multiclass outlier classification with MapReduce framework.

The a priori method of MapReduce structure and association rule can be used to identify the relationship between a disease and its symptoms.

The experiment was done by collecting the data from UCI machine learning datasets of diabetes comprising 50 attributes and the results of the abovementioned methodology are evaluated by the parameters precision, accuracy, recall, and F1-score [24].

The overall goal of the study is to identify diabetes based on data and provide the best outcome for patients.

The procedure of this hierarchical technique is described below.

3.29.2 Methodology of Hierarchical Technique

The overall method is shown in Figure 3.9.

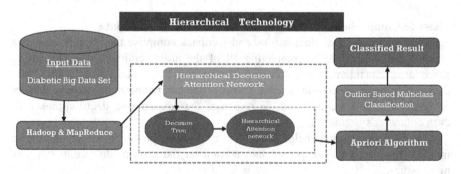

FIGURE 3.9 Hierarchical technology is shown through pictures.

Fundamentals and Technicalities of Big Data and Analytics

Step 1: Hadoop and MapReduce

To begin with, MapReduce framework (MRF) is employed as the diabetes dataset is too big. The MapReduce has a mapper function and reducer function, which reduces the voluminous data without losing of any significant information.

The dataset in the form of diabetes.csv is given as input to the mapper function. Every record in this case has a particular number of fields or characteristics extracted from it. On key value setup, the MRF is embedded and receives the input. As output, the mapper divides the mined data into key–value pairs. The documentation is processed in parallel, producing pairs of key–value data that are equal in Eq. (3.1). The reducer phase uses the result of this phase as an input.

$$\text{Map}(key1, value1) \rightarrow \text{list}(key2, value2) \qquad (3.1)$$

Conversely, the reduce step creates text key–value pairs to match. The result of the reduction step is the union of all intermediate values, which are then organised for processing and often into key–value pairs. The output obtained is well-organised as in Eq. (3.2):

$$\text{Reduce}(key2, \text{list}(value2)) \rightarrow \text{list}(key3, value3) \qquad (3.2)$$

The processing of MRF is depicted in Figure 3.10. A large dataset is split into smaller datasets with different features using MapReduce. The reduced data are used for further processing.

Step 2: Network algorithm for decisions and hierarchical attention (HDAN)

The output of MapReduce step is provided to the HDAN. This network comprises of a hierarchy of a DT, hierarchical attention network (HAN).

- **Decision Tree (DT)**

A DT algorithm is a supervised algorithm suitable for classifying categorical data by their attributes. In data mining, the Map-Reduce data are represented as in Eq. (3.3):

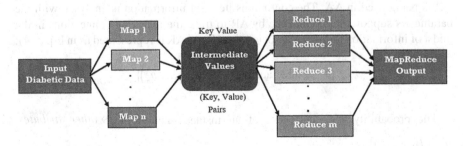

FIGURE 3.10 Map-reduce framework.

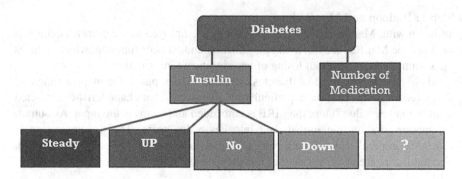

FIGURE 3.11 Decision tree classifier.

$$(u,V) = (u_1, u_2, u_3, \ldots, u_n, V) \tag{3.3}$$

The target feature V must be classified using input variables or features such as u_1, u_2, u_3, etc., represented by the vector u.

Figure 3.11 shows the DT classification method. Different characteristics (steady, up, not and down) can be used to detect the presence of insulin. Figure 3.11 illustrates the importance of insulin and the number of drugs.

- **Hierarchical Attention Network (HAN)**

The HAN comprises of an encoder and decoder. The DT results are used by this HAN. The input information is being processed by encoder with the help of Long Short-Term Memory (LSTM). The decoder maps the output of the encoder to the ideal yield with the help of second LSTM (recurrent layer).

The information table is divided into training and test data. At this stage, the text information is converted to numeric sequences and spaces are inserted between the characters. Text normally has different sequence lengths. Due to this, the converted numeric sequences will also have different lengths, so they require padding. The output of decision tree attention network is fed to the next phase a priori algorithm (AA).

Step 3: A priori algorithm
AR is being used in AA. The continuous item set information is analysed with the parameters support and confidence by AR to trace the recurring connections in the midst of information termed as associations. Hence AR is represented as in Eq. (3.4):

$$\{u_1 \rightarrow \text{other attributes from}(u_2, \ldots, u_n)\} \tag{3.4}$$

The probability of occurrences of an instance i.e., $P\{u_1 \rightarrow other\ attributes\ from(u_2, \ldots u_n)\}$ is estimated by support parameter given as in Eq. (3.5):

Fundamentals and Technicalities of Big Data and Analytics

A target is added to continuous items if the support value is greater than or equal to the *minimum_support*.

$$\text{Support} = \frac{\text{No of transactions}}{\text{No of transactions in database}} \quad (3.5)$$

The confidence of the rule $P\{u_1 \rightarrow \text{other attributes from } (u_2,\ldots,u_n)\}$ implies the probability of both predecessor and resultant in an identical operation.

The confidence is represented by Eq. (3.6). If the inference confidence set by the norm is greater than or equal to *minimum_confidence*, then that norm is added to the AR arrangement.

$$\text{Confidence}\{u_1 \rightarrow \text{other attributes from}(u_2,\ldots,u_n)\} = \frac{(u_1 \cup (u_2,\ldots,u_n))}{(u_1)} \quad (3.6)$$

The results acquired from AA are fed to the next stage, multi-class categorisation based on outliers.

Step 4: Multi-class categorisation based on outliers

The output from AA is used as the input in this phase, which is the last step. Here, the output of AA is categorised based on the prediction made using support and confidence scores. The dataset is divided into train and test samples. To identify diabetic patients, first training has been conducted. In order to classify the patient as having diabetes, testing is performed.

Results and observations from simulations

The dataset of UCI ML [25] was used in this work. Initially, this diabetes dataset consists of 50 attributes and 101,767 records and is arranged in Table 3.3.

The experiment was conducted with MapReduce technique with HDAN operations, association rule and multi-class anomaly classification algorithm, and the results are evaluated.

Figure 3.12(a) represents original diabetic dataset has 101,767 records and Figure 3.12(b) count the records of map-reduce results. The given dataset is mapped and then reduced to 20,588 records after applying the MapReduce technique. Thus, a large set of diabetes data is greatly reduced by features.

Figure 3.13 depicts the parallel MapReduce execution. After MapReduce, the dataset's 15 attributes, including age, gender, weight, medical specialisation, length of hospital stay, etc., are processed. Further, a hierarchical decision attention network receives this MapReduce result as input.

The output of the HDAN is depicted in Figure 3.14. The association rule AA is used to analyse diseases, and diabetes individuals need to be given insulin. To assess issues like {insulin} → {diabetes}, ARM is used. Additionally, the confidence value is given as 1, and the support value is given as 0.60.

TABLE 3.3
Diabetes dataset attributes

Attributes in diabetic dataset		
encounter_id	Race	patient_nbr
Gender	Weight	age
admission type id	admission_source_id	discharge disposition id
time_in_hospital	medical_specialty	payer_code
num_procedures	num_lab_procedures	num_medications
number_emergency	number_outpatient	num_inpatient
diag 2	diag_1	diag 3
max_glu_serum	number_diagnoses	AICresult
Nateglinide	repaglinide	Metformin
Acetohexamide	glimepiride	Chlorpropamide
Tolbutamide	glyburide	Glipizide
Acarbose	rosiglitazone	Pioglitazone
troglitazone	Migitol	Tolazamide
citoglipton	Examide	Insulin
glipizide-metformin	glyburide-metformin	glimepiride-pioglitazone
metformin-pioglitazone	metformin-rosiglitazone	Change
readmitted	diabetesMed	

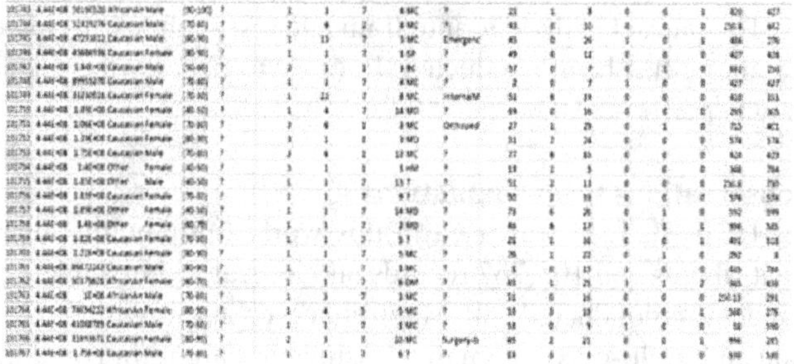

(a): Original diabetic dataset has 101767 records

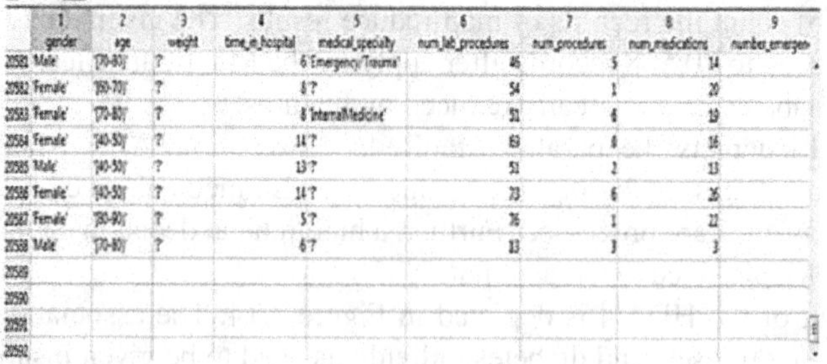

20588d3 table

	1 gender	2 age	3 weight	4 time_in_hospital	5 medical_specialty	6 num_lab_procedures	7 num_procedures	8 num_medications	9 number_emergen
20581	Male'	[70-80)'	?	6	'Emergency/Trauma'	46	5	14	
20582	Female'	[60-70)'	?	8	?	54	1	20	
20583	Female'	[70-80)'	?	8	'InternalMedicine'	51	4	19	
20584	Female'	[40-50)'	?	14	?	63	4	16	
20585	Male'	[40-50)'	?	13	?	51	2	13	
20586	Female'	[40-50)'	?	14	?	73	6	25	
20587	Female'	[80-90)'	?	5	?	76	1	22	
20588	Male'	[70-80)'	?	6	?	13	1	3	
20589									
20590									
20591									
20592									

(b): Dataset record obtained after MapReduce

FIGURE 3.12 (a) Original diabetic dataset has 101767 records. Dataset record obtained after MapReduce.

```
Parallel mapreduce execution on the parallel pool:
**********************************
*        MAPREDUCE PROGRESS       *
**********************************
Map    0%  Reduce    0%
Map   50%  Reduce    0%
Map  100%  Reduce    0%
Map  100%  Reduce  100%
```

FIGURE 3.13   Execution of MapReduce in parallel.

TABLE 3.4
An evaluation of the approaches

Parameters	Hierarchical Algorithm	DT + Apriori + Outlier Multi-class	DT	RBF Network
Precision	0.99	0.99	0.89	0.824
Probability of detection	0.99	0.7	0.65	0.871
F1-score	0.99	0.82	0.73	0.847

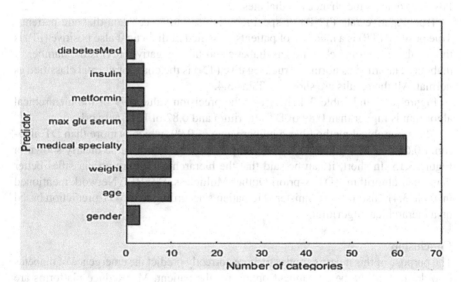

FIGURE 3.14   HDAN results.

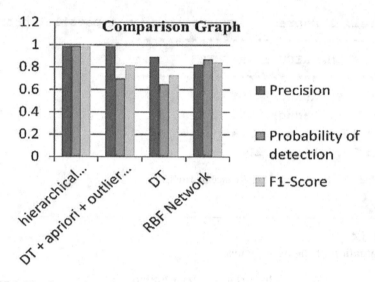

FIGURE 3.15 Comparison chart.

After applying the classification method, they are divided into two categories: diabetics and non-diabetics. Sensitivity, specificity, accuracy, precision and F1score value can be calculated from the confusion matrix. Higher value of "True Positive" detects the chances of diabetes.

True negative rate (TNR) or specificity is used to screen non-diabetic patients. True positive (TP) is a measure of patients classified as diabetic. False positive (FP) is the number of normal classified as diabetic and false negative (FN) is the number of diabetics classified as normal. True Negative (TN) is the count of normal classified as normal. All the results are shown in Table 3.4.

Figure 3.15 and Table 3.4 show that the precision value 0.99 of the hierarchical algorithm is higher than 0.89 of DT algorithm and 0.82 of RBF network.

The hierarchical method has a higher value of 0.99, which is more than DT algorithm 0.65 and RBF network 0.871, compared to the return value clearly shown in Figure 3.15. In short, it can be said that the hierarchical algorithm classifies better than other algorithms (DT A-priori Outlier Multiclass, DT, RBF Network mentioned in Table 3.4). Insulin is administered to patients according to the DT prediction based on a hierarchical algorithm.

Conclusion

The purpose of this investigation is to more correctly predict the emergence of diabetes in order to find the best treatment option for the patient. MapReduce platforms are utilised in association with hierarchical algorithms like HDAN, outlier based multiclass classification, AA to carry out this study. With the help of this, the insulin levels of diabetes patients are identified and categorised. Evidently, the hierarchical approach performs better as seen by the comparison graph. For greater accessibility and real-time performance, this algorithm may also have access to cloud computing resources.

3.30 FUTURE OF BIG DATA IN HEALTHCARE: TECHNICAL CHALLENGES, POSSIBILITIES

Despite the extensive advantages of employing big data analytics, there are drawbacks as well.

3.30.1 BIG DATA CHALLENGES IN HEALTHCARE

Any industry that relies on data faces issues with data administration, tracking, storage, accessibility, prices, and analysis. However, due to the volume of private data generated each day, a big data solution can benefit the healthcare industry. The five V's of big data – velocity, volume, value, variety, and veracity – are crucial to understanding how this industry is tackling and resolving big data difficulties.

3.30.1.1 Velocity Challenge: In Healthcare, Time Is More Crucial than Money

Data velocity refers to how quickly large amounts of data can be created, transmitted, and processed. Making sure all datasets feed into the server quickly and efficiently is the difficulty. Data types such as the main symptoms of patients must be updated in real time, while the maintenance of readmission reports or the speed of patient collection is significantly slower.

Platforms for cloud-based integration can virtually merge disparate databases. Processing data is made quicker and more efficient by carrying out data quality checks and repairs across these linked databases. These platforms also influence clinician decision-making favourably by aiding in the synchronisation of data across clinical systems, which fosters the provision of high-quality patient care.

3.30.1.2 Volume Challenge: More Big Data than Any Other Industry

Particularly in the healthcare sector, the amount of data available is expanding unabatedly. The volume is growing as a result of additional data sources and larger, more complicated databases. Different organisations need to identify systems that handle heavy data without disrupting essential functions such as accessing electronic health records or communicating with a provider.

Big data integration tools make it possible for businesses to migrate big data sets at a reasonable cost and with no need for configuration. Building a global data lake could enable healthcare businesses like AstraZeneca to gain double the value for half the price.

3.30.1.3 Value Challenge: Healthcare Raises the Importance of Data Quality

Whether big data can generate any real and significant return on investment is a key factor in determining its worth. The value derived from analysis depends on specific cases such as revenue reduction, identifying precise patient populations or performance reporting because health data is large and complex.

Value can be found in the form of better outcomes, strategic choices, and increased company efficiencies. Today, it is an organisation that seeks the right understanding of importance and implementation for companies that need to follow management ethics and improve IT principles with qualified data scientists. The costs of poor data quality in this industry can be deadly.

A comprehensive picture of patients can be achieved with the aid of integrated solutions of big data to facilitate intelligence teams in various businesses to search useful trends.

Properly connected big data designed for to identify which patients are about to drop out of their policy within a certain period of time. Timelines for patient assessments can be more effectively planned with the aid of predictive analytics.

Healthcare organisations can utilise these data trends to determine when patients should repeat examinations, and organisations can save time and money by postponing test scheduling.

3.30.1.4 Variety Challenge: There Are Numerous Sources and Forms for Data

The variety of big data sources and types that are available poses a hurdle. Key insights regarding patients and procedures are severely hampered by the constant production of new and varied data forms, contexts, and types.

Additionally, merging big data into conventional databases is challenging due to data sets being located in different places. APIs and latest standards such as Fast Healthcare Interoperability Resources (FHIR) are needed to process data sets that unable to tune by conventional course of action similar to manual preparation or ETL.

Integrating open-source big data technology with proprietary data formats is possible. They can be set up to grow and process more transactions, meet up, or exceed service level agreements (SLAs) for claim processing times and agreement standards, and streamline migration processes that cause no downtime for clients.

3.30.1.5 Veracity Challenge: Authentic Information Is Necessary for Healthcare

Veracity is a problem that concerns the reliability of big data and its conclusions. It is impossible to use insights generated from biased or unreliable data.

As unstructured data inputs undermine data quality, providers always seek to increase data integrity. Healthcare businesses may guarantee standardised, ready, clean, and full data through data governance frameworks and data quality standards.

Users are able to comprehend and interact with the data on their own thanks to cloud data preparation technologies. Healthcare firms can minimise their time to get insight above 50%, allowing them to consume data more quickly and effectively and tailor their messaging to the correct people.

Big Data also creates a number of issues, including difficulty with data collection, storage, processing, and display [26]. Data standardisation (information is put away in groups that are not consistent with all applications and advances), security (information security, privacy, and sensitivity of health data are considered to be important related to confidentiality), and data structure (Big Data should be usable, transparent, and choice-based, but fragmented, distributed, rarely standardised, and

Fundamentals and Technicalities of Big Data and Analytics

difficult to compile and analyse) (health care should be able to use Big Data in real time) [27, 28].

3.30.1.6 Other Challenges
- *Information availability.* Storage and processing become more difficult as data volume increases. Big data must be appropriately kept and preserved such that data scientists and analysts with less experience can use without any hazards.
- *Upkeep of data quality.* Due to the large amount of data received from different sources and in different formats, managing the quality of big data requires a lot of time, effort, and resources to maintain the quality of the data.
- *Protecting data.* The complexity of big data systems creates certain security problems. Properly managing information security issues in the context of a complex big data environment can be challenging.
- *Choosing the appropriate tools.* There is a huge variety of big data analytics platforms and tools available, so it can be difficult for companies to choose the one that best suits their user requirements and infrastructure.
- Some companies are struggling to fill the gaps, due to a lack of internal analytics and the high cost of hiring skilled data scientists and engineers.

3.30.2 HEALTHCARE'S BIG DATA FUTURE AND OPPORTUNITIES

Big data in healthcare has significant potential to transform healthcare, improve patient health, predict disease, provide intuitive information, prevent preventable illnesses, reduce healthcare costs, and generally improve quality of life [29].

Determining the tactics used by medical institutions to encourage and execute such solutions and the benefits of using big data analysis is a topic for future research on the use of big data in medical institutions. There are essentially unlimited opportunities for future healthcare research. These [30, 31] suggest a method that can be applied in various healthcare applications when using big data analytics to diagnose particular illnesses.

Big Data Analytics can also be applied to the outspread of pandemics, the effectiveness of cancer treatment [32, 33] or psychology and psychotherapy research, such as recognition of emotions [34].

The true future of healthcare lies in using these technologies for greater impact, including artificial intelligence, machine learning, and natural language processing. A group of technologies known as artificial intelligence (AI) are able to think and adapt on their own [35, 36]. AI can be used in healthcare to detect illness, set up clinical trial cohorts, and spot malignant tumours, among other things.

Artificial intelligence is divided into machine learning and natural language processing. To describe data, machine learning includes creating models. The algorithms adjust to the new data as it is added to produce models that as closely as possible match the data [35]. With the assistance of machine learning, precision medicine practitioners can determine the best course of treatment for a patient based on their individual medical history.

To understand speech or text produced by humans, natural language processing (NLP) employs a variety of methods [35]. Information extraction from patient data and clinical document classification are two areas where NLP is particularly helpful.

3.31 BIG DATA PERSPECTIVES FOR 2022

The following notable Big Data statistics show the development and importance of this field [37].

A study titled "Big Data Market by Component, Deployment Mode, Organization Size, Business Function (Finance, Marketing & Sales), Industry Vertical (BFSI, Manufacturing, Healthcare & Life Sciences) and Region – Global Forecast to 2026" published by Markets and Markets projects that the market will raise from $162.6 billion in 2021 to $273.4 billion in 2026 at a compound annual growth rate (CAGR) of 11.0% during the estimated period [38].

Interestingly, 99.5% of the data that is gathered is never used or examined. So much untapped potential! Adoption of big data analytics could have a significant positive impact on healthcare. Annual savings of up to $300 billion are possible!

According to statistics, adopting big data can boost retail sales by 3–4%. The demand for tools to process the information grows as more businesses utilise the capabilities of Big Data analytics. The market for big data software is expected to reach $46 billion in 2027, growing at a CAGR of 12.6% [39].

More than 1 billion gigabytes of data are stored on YouTube's servers, which get 300 hours of fresh video every minute [40].

Big data engineers in India make an average of INR 7.88 lakh annually. Depending on their qualifications and expertise, it might range from INR 3.99 lakh to INR 17 lakh annually [41].

According to experts, big data analytics can significantly improve the healthcare sector. According to their estimates, this industry might save up to $300 billion annually by utilising big data [42].

In 2018, software solutions for business intelligence and analytics generated an astounding $24 billion in global revenue [43].

The aforementioned facts make it very evident that the big data sector is expanding quickly. Every day, we produce enormous amounts of data, and businesses understand their value. Therefore, utilising recent Big Data technology [44, 45] can aid numerous industries in accelerating their expansion.

3.32 SUMMARY

In this chapter, we covered an in-depth introduction to big data, including how its V-values (such as volume, variety, and velocity) affect the volume, velocity, and variety of health data. A discussion was also presented related to challenges and issues in big data healthcare. From users' perspective, we described many open source technologies needed to manage this voluminous data. "Data Analytics during the COVID-19 Pandemic" uses the function and importance of big data analytics in healthcare as a case study.

Operational and analytical big data techniques are also covered in this chapter. Four broad areas of big data technologies and techniques are mentioned here. Here we discussed the various stages of big data analysis followed by the healthcare industry.

This chapter includes a case study that uses MapReduce big data to determine whether a patient has diabetes or not. One of the most popular big data frameworks is MapReduce. The core components of the MapReduce programming paradigm are the two user-written procedures Map and Reduce. The map procedure accepts a single key–value pair and creates a list of key–value pairs. A group of transitional values associated with the same intermediate key is transmitted to the Reduce function. The reduce procedure takes as input an array of key and space bar values. It combines these values to reduce the number of numbers. Finally, this chapter talks about the future of big data in healthcare, technical challenges and opportunities.

REFERENCES

[1] Bansal, Ankita, and Niranjan Kumar. "Aspect-Based Sentiment Analysis Using Attribute Extraction of Hospital Reviews." *New Generation Computing* 41, no. 2 (2021): 1–20.

[2] Bhatia, Poonam, and Rajender Nath. "Using Sentiment Analysis in Patient Satisfaction: A Survey." *Advances in Mathematics: Scientific Journal* 9, no. 6 (2020): 3803–3812.

[3] https://archive.physionet.org/mimic2/

[4] www.elderresearch.com/blog/the-42-vs-of-big-data-and-data-science/

[5] Bajaber, Fuad, SherifSakr, Omar Batarfi, Abdulrahman Altalhi, and Ahmed Barnawi. "Benchmarking Big Data Systems: A Survey." *Computer Communications* 149 (2020): 241–251.

[6] Ghosh, Partha. "Deep Learning to Diagnose Diseases and Security in 5G Healthcare Informatics." In *Machine Learning and Deep Learning Techniques for Medical Science*, pp. 279–331. CRC Press, 2022. DOI: 10.1201/9781003217497-16

[7] Pham, Quoc-Viet, Dinh C. Nguyen, Thien Huynh-The, Won-Joo Hwang, and Pubudu N. Pathirana. "Artificial intelligence (AI) and Big Data for Coronavirus (COVID-19) Pandemic: A Survey on the State-of-the-Arts." *IEEE Access* 8 (2020): 130820.

[8] Ghosh, P., and S. Ghosh. "IoT And Machine Learning in Green Smart Home Automation and Green Building Management." *Journal of Alternate Energy and Source Technology* 10, no. 3 (2020): 8–36.

[9] https://martech.zone/benefits-of-big-data/

[10] Guraya, Salman Y. "Transforming Laparoendoscopic Surgical Protocols During the COVID-19 Pandemic; Big Data Analytics, Resource Allocation and Operational Considerations." *International Journal of Surgery* 80 (2020): 21–25.

[11] Rahmanti, AnnisaRistya, Dina Nur Anggraini Ningrum, Lutfan Lazuardi, Hsuan-Chia Yang, and Yu-Chuan Jack Li. "Social Media Data Analytics for Outbreak Risk Communication: Public Attention on the 'New Normal' During the COVID-19 Pandemic in Indonesia." *Computer Methods and Programs in Biomedicine* 205 (2021): 106083.

[12] Wang, Yiting, Ting Wang, Ying Cui, Honghui Mei, Xiao Wen, Jinzhi Lu, and Wei Chen. "COVID-19 Data Visualization Public Welfare Activity." *Visual Informatics* 4, no. 3 (2020): 51–54.

[13] Çallı, Erdi, EcemSogancioglu, Bram van Ginneken, Kicky G. van Leeuwen, and Keelin Murphy. "Deep Learning for Chest X-ray Analysis: A Survey." *Medical Image Analysis* 72 (2021): 102125.

[14] www.seagate.com/files/www-content/our-story/trends/files/idc-seagate-dataage-whitepaper.pdf

[15] Prasad, Bakshi Rohit, and Sonali Agarwal. "Comparative Study of Big Data Computing and Storage Tools: A Review." *International Journal of Database Theory and Application* 9, no. 1 (2016): 45–66.

[16] Salloum, Salman, Ruslan Dautov, Xiaojun Chen, Patrick Xiaogang Peng, and Joshua Zhexue Huang. "Big Data Analytics on Apache Spark." *International Journal of Data Science and Analytics* 1, no. 3 (2016): 145–164.

[17] Bergamaschi, Sonia, Luca Gagliardelli, Giovanni Simonini, and Song Zhu. "BigBench Workload Executed by Using Apache Flink." *Procedia Manufacturing* 11 (2017): 695–702.

[18] Ghosh, P., S. Roy, S. Bose, and A. Mondal. "A Survey on Deep Learning based Detection of Abnormal Human Behaviour using Computer Vision Human Activity Recognition System" *Journal of Computer Technology & Applications*, 12(3) (2021): 32–41.

[19] Ghosh, P. "Timely Diabetes Possibility Prediction using AI Techniques," *Journal of Artificial Intelligence Research & Advances*, 9, no. 2 (2022): 37–47.

[20] Ghosh, Partha, Kalyani Mali, and Sitansu Kumar Das. "Chaotic Firefly Algorithm-based Fuzzy C-means Algorithm for Segmentation of Brain Tissues in Magnetic Resonance Images." *Journal of Visual Communication and Image Representation* 54 (2018): 63–79.

[21] Ghosh, Partha, Kalyani Mali, and Sitansu K. Das. "Use of Spectral Clustering Combined with Normalized Cuts (N-Cuts) in an Iterative k-means Clustering Framework (NKSC) for Superpixel Segmentation with Contour Adherence." *Pattern Recognition and Image Analysis* 28, no. 3 (2018): 400–409.

[22] Ghosh, Partha, Kalyani Mali, and S. K. Das. "Superpixel Segmentation with Contour Adherence Using Spectral Clustering, Combined with Normalized Cuts (N-Cuts) in an Iterative k-means Clustering Framework (NKSC)." *International Journal of Engineering and Future Technology* 14, no. 3 (2017): 23–37.

[23] Ghosh, P., S. K. Das, and K. Mali. "Comparative Analysis of Proposed FCM Clustering Integrated Enhanced Firefly-optimized Algorithm (En-FAOFCM) for MR Image Segmentation and Performance Evaluation." *Journal of Image Processing and Pattern Recognition Progress* 3 (2016): 32–44.

[24] Jayasri, N. P., and R. Aruna. "Big Data Analytics in Health Care by Data Mining and Classification Techniques." *ICT Express* 8, no. 2 (2022): 250–257.

[25] https://archive.ics.uci.edu/ml/datasets/diabetes

[26] Chen, Hsinchun, Roger HL Chiang, and Veda C. Storey. "Business Intelligence and Analytics: From Big Data to Big Impact." *MIS Quarterly* (2012): 1165–1188.

[27] Bainbridge, Michael. "Big Data Challenges for Clinical and Precision Medicine." In *Big Data, Big Challenges: A Healthcare Perspective*, pp. 17–31. Springer, Cham, 2019.

[28] Ismail, Ahmed, Abdulaziz Shehab, and I. M. El-Henawy. "Healthcare Analysis in Smart Big Data Analytics: Reviews, Challenges and Recommendations." In *Security in Smart Cities: Models, Applications, and Challenges*, pp. 27–45. Springer, Cham, 2019.

[29] Abouelmehdi, Karim, Abderrahim Beni-Hessane, and Hayat Khaloufi. "Big Healthcare Data: Preserving Security and Privacy." *Journal of Big Data* 5, no. 1 (2018): 1–18. doi: 10.1186/s40537-017-0110-7

[30] Shubham, Shubham, Nikita Jain, Vedika Gupta, Senthilkumar Mohan, Mazeyanti MohdAriffin, and Ali Ahmadian. "Identify Glomeruli in Human Kidney Tissue Images Using a Deep Learning Approach." *Soft Computing* (2021): 1–12. doi: 10.1007/s00500-021-06143-z

[31] Willems, Stefan M., SanneAbeln, K. Anton Feenstra, Remco de Bree, Egge F. van der Poel, Robert J. Baatenburg de Jong, JaapHeringa, and Michiel W.M/ van den Brekel. "The Potential Use of Big Data in Oncology." *Oral Oncology* 98 (2019): 8–12. doi: 10.1016/j.oraloncology.2019.09.003

[32] Corsi, Alana, Fabiane Florencio de Souza, Regina Negri Pagani, and JoãoLuiz Kovaleski. "Big Data Analytics as a Tool for Fighting Pandemics: A Systematic Review of Literature." *Journal of Ambient Intelligence and Humanized Computing* 12, no. 10 (2021): 9163–9180. doi: 10.1007/s12652-020-02617-4

[33] Wu, Jun, Jian Wang, Stephen Nicholas, Elizabeth Maitland, and Qiuyan Fan. "Application of Big Data Technology for COVID-19 Prevention and Control in China: Lessons and Recommendations." *Journal of Medical Internet Research* 22, no. 10 (2020): e21980.

[34] Jain, Nikita, Vedika Gupta, Shubham Shubham, AgamMadan, Ankit Chaudhary, and K. C. Santosh. "Understanding Cartoon Emotion Using Integrated Deep Neural Network on Large Dataset." *Neural Computing and Applications* (2021): 1–21. doi: 10.1007/s00521-021-06003-9

[35] Lepenioti, Katerina, Alexandros Bousdekis, Dimitris Apostolou, and Gregoris Mentzas. "Prescriptive Analytics: Literature Review and Research Challenges." *International Journal of Information Management* 50 (2020): 57–70.

[36] Davenport, Thomas, and Ravi Kalakota. "The Potential for Artificial Intelligence in Healthcare." *Future Healthcare Journal* 6, no. 2 (2019): 94.

[37] www.marketsandmarkets.com/Market-Reports/big-data-market-1068.html

[38] www.globenewswire.com/en/news-release/2022/06/08/2458994/0/en/Big-Data-Market-worth-273- 4-billion-by-2026-Report-by-Marketsandmarkets.html

[39] https://webtribunal.net/blog/big-data-stats/#gref

[40] www.disruptordaily.com/7-facts-know-big-data/

[41] www.glassdoor.co.in/Salaries/india-big-data-engineer-salary-SRCH_IL.0,5_IN115_KO6,23.htm

[42] www.gartner.com/en/newsroom

[43] www.statista.com/statistics/551501/worldwide-big-data-business-analytics-revenue/

[44] Seagate. "The Digitization of the World: From Edge to Core," www.seagate.com/files/www-content/our-story/trends/files/idc-seagate-dataage-whitepaper.pdf." Accessed September 29, 2022.

[45] Do It Software. "Top Big Data Technologies in 2022: How They Can Benefit Your Business," https://doit.software/blog/big-data-technologies." Accessed September 29, 2022.

FURTHER READING

Berthold, Michael, David J. Hand, *Intelligent Data Analysis*, Springer-Verlag Berlin and Heidelberg GmbH & Co. KG, ISBN: 9783540430605

Franks, Bill. *Taming the Big Data Tidal Wave*, John Wiley & Sons Inc, ISBN:9781118208786

Leskovec, Jure, Anand Rajaraman, and Jeffrey David Ullman. *Mining of Massive Datasets*, Cambridge University Press, ISBN: 9781316638491

White, Tom. *Hadoop: The Definitive Guide – Storage and Analysis at Internet Scale*, Shroff Publishers & Distributors Pvt Ltd, ISBN: 9789352130672

4 Fundamentals of Health Informatics and Health Data Science

N. S. Prema

4.1 INTRODUCTION

During pregnancy, there can be health problems called pregnancy consequences. They can concern either the mother's or the baby's health, or both. Some women have health issues prior to becoming pregnant that may cause complications. During the pregnancy, other issues arise. The health of either the mother or the foetus may be impacted by these issues. Complications can arise even in women who were in good health before getting pregnant. Due to these issues, the pregnancy can be deemed high-risk (Davis and Narayan 2020).

Females with the past of difficult pregnancies either or both deliveries, as well as diseases like diabetes, immunologic complaints and hypertension, are at a greater risk of having a high-risk pregnancy. Obstetricians/physicians or healthcare workers interpret and classify data based on their expertise and the results of clinical and diagnostic studies; the process is very subjective and requires explaining skills (Gorthi, Firtion, and Vepa 2009; Tonei 2019).

Healthcare industry today generates a large amount of complex data about patience, recourses of hospitals, medical records, devices etc. The amount of data is the main source to process and to analyse in order to extract the knowledge to support cost-savings and decision making (Patil, Joshi, and Toshniwal 2010).

Maternal well-being alludes to women's well-being during the time periods of conception, childbirth, and postpartum. It incorporates the health measures of family planning services, prejudice, childbirth, and postpartum care to promise an encouraging and sufficient involvement with utmost cases and to diminish maternal grimness and mortality in different cases.

The ability to detect and predict early pregnancy complications allows for better controlling and outcomes including both mother and child, enabling medical professionals to work more efficiently in resource provision and provide apt response to a variety of medical complications.

4.2 C-SECTION DELIVERY (CS)

There are numerous myths surrounding the delivery method during pregnancy. According to clinical scientists, accurately predicting the childbirth mode remains difficult. On the other hand, early detection or prediction of the delivery mode could help to lessen the worry and stress that comes with it. There are primarily two types of childbirth: C-section and normal or vaginal delivery. A caesarean delivery is an operating procedure that involves delivering a foetus through a cut done in the mother's abdomen and uterus. In mammals, vaginal delivery is the natural method of birth. Although both methods of delivery are common, caesarean deliveries come with risks and problems, such as infection, haemorrhage, blood clots, and so on. It also involves pain control, financial, and other preparedness.

It is universally accepted in safe motherhood strategies that providing crucial obstetric care and ensuring institutional delivery are the best choices for reducing maternal mortality in every circumstances. Institutional delivery allows for the resolution of delivery complications.

In these conditions, the amount of all caesarean deliveries are taken as a sign to measure problems and recognize access to excellence in obstetric care in various populations. Because it doesn't represent quality care, but rather expresses an unhealthy trend both in medical profession and society (Masukume et al. 2019).

As a result, the rising drift in caesarean births suggests that this practice is being used for reasons other than maternal complications. It also endangers the mother's health and wastes resources. According to UNICEF, WHO, and UNFPA guidelines, at least 5% of deliveries will require a caesarean section to save the life of the mother or the infant. The World Health Organization commends that caesarean delivery rates not surpass 15% in general. Rates greater than 15% indicate improper use of the procedure.

As against this, the current level of caesarean delivery in many countries is as high as 30–50%. The rising trend is highest in the United States and in some countries like Brazil and Mexico in Latin America. The percentage of caesarean deliveries in the United States is drastically increasing over the years. According to current data, 1.2 million or 29.1% of all births took place in the United States are via C-Section in 2004 (NIHS, 2006).

Even in an evolving country India, there is a growing fashion of C-Section delivery, as institutional deliveries increase and the availability of obstetric and gynaecological care increases. According to an Indian Council of Medical Research (ICMR) study, the average caesarean section rate in 33 tertiary care institutions increased from 21.8% in 1993–1994 to 25.4% in 1998–1999 (Das, Devi, and Kim 2014). According to the National Family Health Survey, 1992–1993, Kerala and Goa had the maximum percentage of C-Section deliveries (Mishra and Ramanathan 2002).

Over the last ten years, where both excess use and unmet demand are anticipated to co-occur, use of C-Section has increased gradually throughout the world. Southern Asia and Sub-Saharan Africa will face a complex situation with morbidity and mortality linked to unmet needs, unsafe C-Section provision, and concurrent overuse of the surgical procedure that depletes resources and increases avoidable morbidity and mortality when effective global actions are lacking to reverse the trend. To fulfil the Sustainable Development Goals, there should be a global focus on fully resolving the C-Section issue (Betran et al. 2021).

TABLE 4.1
The major risk factors associated with caesarean delivery

Socio-demographic	• Maternal age at delivery • Women's lifestyle: smoking, alcohol consumption, drug use, stress, and so on. • Social class of the mother • Profession
Medical	• Had varicose veins • Had haemorrhoids/piles • Had convulsions/fever • Foetal presentation
Obstetric history	• Previous caesarean section • Outcome of last pregnancy like child alive, miscarriage/termination, and stillbirth/child died etc. • Inter-pregnancy interval • Parity
Antenatal history	• Hypertension • Diabetes mellitus

There are three types of risks associated with caesarean delivery: short-term risks, long-term risks, and risks related to future pregnancies. There are also risks to the newborn that must be taken into account. Certainly, the clinical situation that leads to a caesarean delivery has a major impact on the possibility of complications (Keag, Norman, and Stock 2018; Sandall et al. 2018).

The perceived risk also differs significantly between a primary caesarean section performed on an average-weight woman who is not in labour and an emergency caesarean section performed on an obese woman who has been in labour for hours. In a similar vein, when interpreting studies on the risk of caesarean delivery, it is important to remember that comparing women who delivered by caesarean with those who delivered normally may not be appropriate. Most studies attempt to distinguish between women who had planned caesarean deliveries and those who had caesarean sections during labour in order to compare situations of similarity rather than contrast. Although research has not been definitive, C-Section has repeatedly been linked to a higher risk of obesity later in life (Masukume et al. 2018; Chiavarini et al. 2021; Cavalcante et al. 2022; Young et al. 2018). The major risk factors of caesarean delivery are shown in Table 4.1.

4.3 DEMOGRAPHIC AND SOCIOECONOMIC

Maternal age and race are the main demographic factors linked to preterm birth risk that are frequently seen. Extreme maternal ages are characteristics that lead to low birth weight births and pulmonary tuberculosis. These illnesses are more likely to complicate pregnancies in adolescent women. Due to pre-existing illnesses and the development of new ones, women over 40 have an even higher risk of developing these conditions (Behrman and Butler 2007).

Race is thought to have an impact on maternal health. Several research models show that when compared to native white women, African American women have a greater threat of preterm birth. Additionally, studies have shown a connection between pregnancy problems and low socioeconomic position, poor educational rank, and single motherhood (Goldenberg et al. 2008, Valdes 2021).

4.4 RELATED WORK

The following are the some of the work carried out by the researchers in predicting the type of delivery.

Decision tree induction based prediction model is proposed for the detection of type of delivery using pregnancy characteristics. The model achieved an accuracy of 84% in C-Section and vaginal delivery prediction (Pereira et al. 2015). Further application of decision tree is also shown for the determination of type delivery with a highest accuracy of 86% (Gharehchopogh, Mohammadi, and Hakimi 2012).

A priori association rule has been used for mining the association between the caesarean delivery and high heart rate, high blood pressure, and low education levels. They have also prepared a prediction model using decision tree and neural network for the prediction of the type of the delivery (Sana, Razzaq, and Ferzund 2012). Based on the data obtained from ultrasonography reports, urine, and blood test reports, prediction of mode of delivery is done using ID3 and Naïve Bayes classifier (Kamat, Oswal, and Datar 2015).

Sunantha Sodsee has suggested a nearest neighbours (NN) algorithm based on the cephalopelvic disproportion (CPD) to predict caesarean deliveries. In the suggested NN, nearest and farthest neighbours are determined using two threshold distances. The suggested model achieves the highest performance (Sodsee, 2014).

A classification model was prepared that allow an estimate of the range for the Apgar score value depending on the mother, new born data. They have proposed tool for the prediction and analysis of type of birth using different classification models (Robu and Holban 2015).

To help doctors make the best decisions, Abbas et al. presented a decision support system employing machine learning procedures. For the examination of C-Section delivery risk factors, they have used Naïve Bayes, neural networks, support vector machine (SVM) and k-nearest neighbour (kNN) classifiers (Abbas et al. 2018). To assess and predict in vitro fertilization (IVF) pregnancy more accurately, Md Rafiul Hassan et al. suggested an attribute selection method combined with automatic categorization utilizing machine learning techniques. We evaluated their usage of five attributes, five distinct approaches of machine learning, including SVM, MLP, C4.5, Random Forest and CART, to predict the likelihood of an IVF pregnancy (Hassan et al. 2020).

In two areas in rural southern Ghana, the work targeted to determine the prevalence of caesarean sections and factors that may be related to them. Caesarean section rates are correlated with the mother's age, parity, education level, socioeconomic position of the family, district of habitation, and degree of education of the household head (Manyeh et al. 2018).

In private healthcare facilities, women in Punjab were more expected to give birth via C-Section, and there was little distinction between urban and rural areas. The risk of C-Section varied significantly across the divisions of Punjab, with DG Khan and Rawalpindi showing the lowest risk when matched to the reference division of Bahawalpur. This variation in risk can be partially attributed to the gaps in development and accessibility to public healthcare facilities. The management should make it easier for people, especially rural women, to obtain healthcare facilities in easily accessible locations (Abbas, Amir ud Din, and Sadiq 2018).

The shift in the C-Section rate between 1998 and 2017 in Indonesia was examined, along with the socioeconomic, regional, and health system aspects that may have contributed to it. In order to investigate the factors that influence the utilization of C-sections, researchers ran bivariate and multivariate logistic regressions. In Indonesia, the C-Section rate has gradually risen during the previous 20 years. The rising use of C-sections was linked to factors in the women's socioeconomic level and the health care system (Wyatt et al. 2021).

Higher probabilities of repeated C-Section delivery were found for Hispanic and Black women than with white women after parity adjustments and the application of induction or augmentation techniques. These results were unaffected by anthropometric or demographic variables. Our result highlights the necessity to investigate risk variables beyond those that have been covered in the literature up to this point, which is the first step in developing public health policies and initiatives that target potentially preventable repeated C-Section delivery (Mirabal-Beltran and Strobino, 2020).

In this work, we tried to analyse the effect of demographic and socioeconomic factors on deciding the mode of delivery with the help of statistical tools. We also applied some machine learning techniques for the prediction of mode of delivery with available features.

4.5 EXPERIMENTAL METHODS AND MATERIALS

4.5.1 Background

This section provides the basic concepts of classifiers,

4.5.1.1 Classification

It is a supervised technique of categorizing of object into diverse labelled classes. Naive Bayes, Random Forest, logistic regression, and k-closest neighbour classifier are the classifiers utilized in this study.

Random Forest: The Random Forest algorithm creates the ensemble of the decision tree with the use of the random vector sampled from the decision tree. The decision tree present in the Random Forest contains the input vector and from the input vector, random samples are chosen for the construction of the Random Forest classifier.

Naïve Bayes: It is a probabilistic procedure which uses Bayes rule along with a strong independence assumption forms the basis for Naïve Bayes classifiers. In these classifiers, a simplifying conditional independence assumption is used. Due to this, the class labels like true or false are conditionally independent of each other. Such an assumption makes the classifiers enhance their efficiency and this characteristic is best suited in medical diagnosis.

Logistic regression: It is used to predict outcomes such as this or that, yes or no, A or B, and so on. Although logistic regression can be used for multiclass classification, we will concentrate on this technique's most straightforward use. For binary classifications, it is one of the most widely used machine learning methods.

Nearest neighbour: It is among the earliest prediction methods. The method searches for records with input attributes that are the most comparable in the historical dataset to produce the best prediction, and it then offers the closest value or class of the target variable for this collection of input attributes (Thearling, 2010).

4.5.1.2 Data set

The data set used for the study is linked to maternal healthcare; the data is all about the details of pregnant women. The dataset taken for the study is Pregnancy Risk Assessment Monitoring System (PRAMS) data.

The Centers for Disease Control (CDC) in Atlanta collects data for the PRAMS database, a national database with 32 participating American states. Combining population-based, state-specific sampling, the CDC created the PRAMS database in 1987. Information is gathered on maternal and infant behaviour as well as prenatal, postpartum, and birth experiences (CDC, 2009). It is used to observe the change in indicators of mother and child health and is intended to enhance information from vital records. Parents fill out the questionnaire after the baby is born; it includes pre-, during-, and post-partum behaviour-related questions. The PRAMS database combines information from birth certificates (taken at the moment of birth) and the PRAMS questionnaire (gathered a few months following delivery). The first step in the PRAMS data gathering process is a mail-in survey that is sent two to four months following birth. A telephone interview is used to follow up with non-responders (CDC, 2009).

The data set used for our study is for the year 2015 collected across 34 states. The attributes in the data set includes socio-demographic, medical parameters, obstetric history, antenatal history and some paternal parameters. The analysis of data set is done only with the relevant selected attributes. Most of the attribute values are categorical, very few are continuous.

In this study, the main focus is on the consequence of socio-demographic parameters on the mode of delivery; so we have selected a subset of relevant attributes from the complete dataset. The different modes of delivery considered are first-time C-Section, vaginal delivery, forceps delivery, vacuum delivery, repeated c-section, and vaginal delivery after c-Section. The final data set taken for study contains about 45,000 instances with 49 attributes. The distribution of different modes of delivery is shown in Figure 4.1.

Fundamentals of Health Informatics and Health Data Science

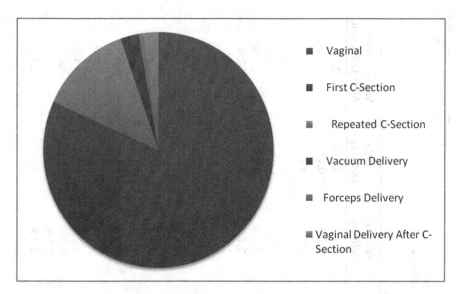

FIGURE 4.1 Distribution of different mode delivery in PRAMS data set.

4.5.2 DEMOGRAPHIC AND SOCIOECONOMIC RISK FACTORS

The percentages of different deliveries for few demographic parameters are tabulated in Table 4.2.

The lists of attributes considered are as follows:

- Ethnicity
- Urban/rural
- Marital status
- Education
- Race
- Smoking
- Alcohol consumption
- Depression
- Abuse
- Body mass index
- Mother's age
- Sex of the baby
- Weight of the baby

4.5.3 DATA PREPARATION

Following the selection of the data, a pre-processing phase was carried out, which included the deletion of data containing nil or noise, leaving 21,400 records for use by the machine learning models. It was also important to assess the dataset with various display of the target variable in light of the expanding machine learning process in

TABLE 4.2
The percentage of different types of delivery for a few socio-demographic parameters

		Delivery Type					
Parameter		Vaginal	First C-Section	Repeated C-Section	Vacuum Delivery	Forceps Delivery	Vaginal Delivery After C-Section
Hispanic	Non-Hispanic	61.4%	20.7%	12.6%	2.6%	0.7%	2.1%
	Hispanic	60.8%	18.9%	15.0%	2.3%	0.4%	2.6%
Urban/Rural	Urban	61.9%	20.2%	12.6%	2.3%	0.7%	2.2%
	Rural	59.9%	20.9%	13.6%	3.2%	0.6%	1.9%
Maternal education	0-8 Years	60.4%	17.3%	16.0%	2.5%	0.4%	3.3%
	9-11 Years	64.2%	16.8%	13.9%	2.5%	0.4%	2.3%
	12 Years	62.5%	18.8%	13.6%	2.4%	0.5%	2.2%
	13-15 Years	60.2%	21.2%	13.9%	2.1%	0.5%	2.2%
	>= 16 Years	60.7%	22.2%	11.0%	3.2%	0.9%	1.9%
Married	Married	60.6%	20.1%	13.7%	2.6%	0.8%	2.2%
	Other	62.4%	21.0%	11.7%	2.5%	0.4%	2.0%
MAT_RACE	Oth Asian	56.9%	24.0%	10.8%	4.5%	1.8%	1.9%
	White	61.7%	20.6%	12.3%	2.6%	0.7%	2.2%
	Black	60.0%	20.4%	14.9%	1.9%	0.3%	2.4%
	Am Indian	63.5%	19.1%	13.1%	2.8%	0.3%	1.2%
	Chinese	64.9%	17.1%	10.4%	5.6%	1.2%	0.8%
	Japanese	74.5%	14.9%	2.1%	4.3%	0.0%	4.3%
	Filipino	55.6%	23.9%	11.1%	6.0%	0.0%	3.4%
	Hawaiian	50.0%	25.0%	25.0%	0.0%	0.0%	0.0%
	Oth-Nonwht	61.8%	17.3%	16.5%	2.2%	0.8%	1.5%
	Ak Native	62.5%	20.0%	12.6%	2.9%	0.7%	1.3%

MOMSMOKE	Yes	59.5 %	19.6 %	15.9 %	2.1 %	0.5 %	2.5 %
	No	61.5 %	20.5 %	12.6 %	2.6 %	0.7 %	2.1 %
INCOME7	$ 0 to $15,000	63.2 %	19.2 %	12.5 %	2.6 %	0.5 %	2.0 %
	$15,001 to $19,000	61.6 %	19.6 %	13.5 %	2.4 %	0.5 %	2.4 %
	$19,001 to $22,000	61.4 %	20.7 %	13.6 %	2.0 %	0.5 %	1.7 %
	$22,001 to $26,000	60.8 %	20.9 %	13.6 %	2.3 %	0.4 %	2.1 %
	$26,001 to $29,000	60.5 %	19.8 %	14.1 %	2.4 %	0.8 %	2.4 %
	$29,001 to $37,000	63.9 %	17.1 %	14.1 %	2.7 %	0.4 %	1.8 %
	$37,001 to $44,000	63.6 %	20.7 %	11.6 %	1.9 %	0.4 %	1.9 %
	$44,001 to $52,000	59.7 %	20.3 %	14.0 %	2.5 %	0.6 %	2.9 %
	$52,001 to $56,000	59.5 %	19.8 %	15.3 %	3.1 %	0.3 %	1.9 %
	$56,001 to $67,000	61.1 %	21.5 %	13.0 %	2.4 %	0.8 %	1.2 %
	$67,001 to $79,000	60.1 %	20.5 %	11.6 %	3.3 %	1.3 %	3.1 %
	$79,001 or more	59.5 %	22.3 %	12.4 %	2.8 %	0.8 %	2.1 %
	$ 0 to $15,000	56.8 %	25.0 %	12.0 %	1.6 %	1.6 %	3.1 %
	$15,001 to $19,000	48.1 %	32.1 %	14.8 %	2.5 %	0.0 %	2.5 %

TABLE 4.3
Different groups of the target variables

S. No	Approach	Number of classes	Target
1	Basic	6	1. Vaginal 2. First C-Section 3. Repeated C-Section 4. Vacuum Delivery 5. Forceps Delivery 6. Vaginal Delivery After C-Section
2	Normal Vs Instrumental	2	1. Vaginal +Vaginal Delivery After C-Section 2. First C-Section+ Repeated C-Section + Vacuum Delivery +Forceps Delivery
3	Most frequent Vs less	2	1. Vaginal + First C-Section+ Repeated C-Section 2. Vacuum Delivery +Forceps Delivery+ Vaginal Delivery After C-Section
4	Vaginal Vs C-Section	2	1. Vaginal +Vaginal Delivery After C-Section+ Vacuum Delivery +Forceps Delivery 2. First C-Section+ Repeated C-Section.
5	First C-section versus repeated C-section	2	1. First C-Section 2. Repeated C-Section

order to obtain improved outcomes. Table 4.3 lists all of the approaches that have been tried.

4.6 PROPOSED SYSTEM

Following is the algorithm for our suggested model:

Algorithm: Type of delivery prediction by using classification techniques
Input: PRAMS dataset
Output: Classify dataset into different delivery types
Step 1: Load the dataset.
Step 2: Remove the irrelevant, null and missing value features.
Step 3: Prepare the data for different approaches.
Step 4: Apply the classifiers.
Step 5: Evaluate the performance the models.
Models are evaluated in terms of accuracy.
Accuracy is equal to the ratio of correctly categorized objects to all the objects in the test set.
To separate training and testing data, cross-validation is performed.

TABLE 4.4
Performance measures of the classifiers for the basic approach

Model	AUC	Accuracy	F1	Precision	Recall
KNN	0.60	0.62	0.53	0.51	0.62
Random Forest	0.60	0.60	0.53	0.51	0.60
Naive Bayes	0.65	0.62	0.54	0.53	0.62
Logistic Regression	0.65	0.63	0.52	0.53	0.63

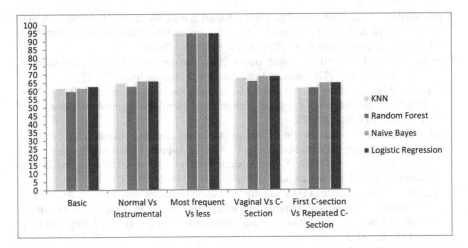

FIGURE 4.2 Accuracy obtained by the models for different approaches.

4.7 RESULTS AND DISCUSSION

The above-mentioned classifiers are applied for the data considering all the attributes, and the algorithms results are shown in Table 4.4. Various classifiers are employed for the prediction; first Random Forest was applied by taking around 10 trees, with five split instances as the maximum. The value of k used for the k-nearest neighbour classifier is 15 and the distances measures used are Euclidean. The classifiers are evaluated using a cross-validation of 10-fold. The performances of the classifiers are presented in Table 4.4. For both sets of data, logistic regression classifier had the highest accuracy. The models are applied for different approaches; the accuracy obtained is shown in Figure 4.2.

4.8 CONCLUSION

The prediction of mode of delivery with the help of machine learning with available limited features will help both medical attenders and patients to take a few precautions; here we have presented a decision support system using which the mode of delivery can be predicted both in first time mothers and repeated pregnancy cases.

The logistic regression classifier has given a highest accuracy of 63%. Our analysis also shows that socio-demographic parameters influence mode of delivery. The data is imbalanced and the ratio of negative classes are more matched to the positive instances. So still there is more scope to increase the classification accuracy by managing imbalanced dataset problem.

REFERENCES

Abbas, Faisal, Rafi Amir ud Din, and Maqsood Sadiq. 2018. "Prevalence and determinants of Caesarean delivery in Punjab, Pakistan." *Eastern Mediterranean Health Journal* 24 (11):1058–1065.

Abbas, Syed Ali, Rabia Riaz, Syed Zaki Hassan Kazmi, Sanam Shahla Rizvi, and Se Jin Kwon. 2018. "Cause analysis of caesarian sections and application of machine learning methods for classification of birth data." *IEEE Access* 6:67555–67561.

Behrman, Richard E, and Adrienne Stith Butler. 2007. *Preterm Birth: Causes, Consequences, and Prevention*. Vol. 772: National Academies Press, Washington, DC.

Betran, Ana Pilar, Jiangfeng Ye, Ann-Beth Moller, João Paulo Souza, and Jun Zhang. 2021. "Trends and projections of caesarean section rates: global and regional estimates." *BMJ Global Health* 6 (6):e005671.

Cavalcante, Lilian Fernanda Pereira, Carolina Abreu de Carvalho, Luana Lopes Padilha, Poliana Cristina de Almeida Fonseca Viola, Antônio Augusto Moura da Silva, and Vanda Maria Ferreira Simões. 2022. "Cesarean section and body mass index in children: is there a causal effect?" *Cadernos de Saúde Pública* 38:e00344020.

Chiavarini, Manuela, Benedetta De Socio, Irene Giacchetta, and Roberto Fabiani. 2021. "Birth by Caesarean section and offspring overweight and obesity in adult life: A systematic review and meta-analysis." *Nutrition and Dietetics Journal* 23 (4):75–84. https://doi.org/10.1111/obr.13423

Das, Rabindra Nath, Rajkumari Sanatombi Devi, and Jinseog Kim. 2014. "Mothers' lifestyle characteristics impact on her neonates' low birth weight." *International Journal of Women's Health and Reproduction Sciences* 2 (4):229–235.

Davis, Elysia Poggi, and Angela J. Narayan. 2020. "Pregnancy as a period of risk, adaptation, and resilience for mothers and infants." *Development and Psychopathology* 32 (5):1625–1639.

Gharehchopogh, Farhad Soleimanian, Peyman Mohammadi, and Parvin Hakimi. 2012. "Application of decision tree algorithm for data mining in healthcare operations: a case study." *International Journal of Computer Applications* 52 (6):21–26.

Goldenberg, Robert L., Jennifer F. Culhane, Jay D. Iams, and Roberto Romero. 2008. "Epidemiology and causes of preterm birth." *The Lancet* no. 371 (9606):75–84.

Gorthi, Aparna, Celine Firtion, and Jithendra Vepa. 2009. Automated risk assessment tool for pregnancy care. Paper read at 2009 Annual International Conference of the IEEE Engineering in Medicine and Biology Society.

Hassan, Md Rafiul, Sadiq Al-Insaif, M. Imtiaz Hossain, and Joarder Kamruzzaman. 2020. "A machine learning approach for prediction of pregnancy outcome following IVF treatment." *Neural Computing and Applications* 32 (7):2283–2297.

Kamat, Alisha, Veenal Oswal, and Manalee Datar. 2015. "Implementation of classification algorithms to predict mode of delivery." *International Journal of Computer Science and Information Technologies* 6 (5):4531–4534.

Keag, Oonagh E., Jane E. Norman, and Sarah J. Stock. 2018. "Long-term risks and benefits associated with cesarean delivery for mother, baby, and subsequent pregnancies: systematic review and meta-analysis." *PLoS Medicine* 15 (1):e1002494.

Manyeh, Alfred Kwesi, Alberta Amu, David Etsey Akpakli, John Williams, and Margaret Gyapong. 2018. "Socioeconomic and demographic factors associated with caesarean section delivery in Southern Ghana: evidence from INDEPTH Network member site." *BMC Pregnancy and Childbirth* 18 (1):1–9.

Masukume, Gwinyai, Fergus P. McCarthy, Philip N. Baker, Louise C. Kenny, Susan M.B. Morton, Deirdre M. Murray, Jonathan O'B. Hourihane, and Ali S. Khashan. 2019. "Association between caesarean section delivery and obesity in childhood: a longitudinal cohort study in Ireland." *BMJ Open* 9 (3):e025051.

Masukume, Gwinyai, Sinéad M. O'Neill, Philip N. Baker, Louise C. Kenny, Susan Morton, and Ali S. Khashan. 2018. "The impact of caesarean section on the risk of childhood overweight and obesity: new evidence from a contemporary cohort study." *Scientific Reports* 8 (1):1–9.

Mirabal-Beltran, Roxanne, and Donna M. Strobino. 2020. "Birth mode after primary cesarean among Hispanic and non-Hispanic women at one US institution." *Women's Health Issues* 30 (1):7–15.

Mishra, Uday S., and Mala Ramanathan. 2002. "Delivery-related complications and determinants of caesarean section rates in India." *Health Policy and Planning* 17 (1):90–98.

Patil, Bankat M., Ramesh Chandra Joshi, and Durga Toshniwal. 2010. "Hybrid prediction model for type-2 diabetic patients." *Expert Systems with Applications* 37 (12):8102–8108.

Pereira, Sónia, Filipe Portela, Manuel Filipe Santos, José Machado, and António Abelha. 2015. "Predicting type of delivery by identification of obstetric risk factors through data mining." *Procedia Computer Science* 64:601–609.

Robu, Raul, and Ştefan Holban. 2015. "The analysis and classification of birth data." *Acta Polytechnica Hungarica* 12 (4):77–96.

Sana, Ayesha, Saad Razzaq, and Javed Ferzund. 2012. "Automated diagnosis and cause analysis of cesarean section using machine learning techniques." *International Journal of Machine Learning and Computing* 2 (5):677.

Sandall, Jane, Rachel M. Tribe, Lisa Avery, Glen Mola, Gerard H.A. Visser, Caroline S.E. Homer, Deena Gibbons, Niamh M. Kelly, Holly Powell Kennedy, and Hussein Kidanto. 2018. "Short-term and long-term effects of caesarean section on the health of women and children." *The Lancet* 392 (10155):1349–1357.

Sodsee, Sunantha. 2014. "Predicting caesarean section by applying nearest neighbor analysis." *Procedia Computer Science* 31:5–14.

Thearling, Kurt. http://thearling.com/ 2010.

Tonei, Valentina. 2019. "Mother's mental health after childbirth: does the delivery method matter?" *Journal of Health Economics* 63:182–196.

Valdes, Elise G. 2021. "Examining cesarean delivery rates by race: a population-based analysis using the Robson Ten-Group Classification System." *Journal of Racial and Ethnic Health Disparities* 8 (4):844–851.

Wyatt, Sage, Permata Imani Ima Silitonga, Esty Febriani, and Qian Long. 2021. "Socioeconomic, geographic and health system factors associated with rising C-section rate in Indonesia: a cross-sectional study using the Indonesian demographic and health surveys from 1998 to 2017." *BMJ Open* 11 (5):e045592.

Young, Carmen B., Shiliang Liu, Giulia M. Muraca, Yasser Sabr, Tracy Pressey, Robert M. Liston, and K.S. Joseph. 2018. "Mode of delivery after a previous cesarean birth, and associated maternal and neonatal morbidity." *CMAJ* 190 (18):E556–E564.

5 Introduction to Disease Prediction

K. V. H. Avani, Deeksha Manjunath and
C. Gururaj

5.1 INTRODUCTION

Agriculture is an important domain with extensive research. The global population is increasing exponentially. To cater to the needs of this increasing population density, agricultural production has to increase in the most effective way. On the negative side, the agriculture field faces the most difficult challenges. Some of the challenges include the cutback of the cultivable land when we require extensive agricultural production. Another greatest challenge is the erratic nature of the climate. As the farmers are completely reliant on the weather for the cultivation of crops, any change in the climate directly affects the production and quality of the cultivating crops.

Weeds are unfavorable plants that thrive on the field lands undesirably that directly affect the quality and production of the edible crops cultivated. Weeds' numerous methods of interfering with crop development and crop culture lead to a reduction in agricultural yields. Weeds impede agricultural cultivation operations by competing with crops for one or more plant growth ingredients, such as nutrients including minerals, water, an energy such as that of sun and expanse. Weeds quickly overrun the crops and use up a lot of water and nutrients because of their hardiness and robust growth habits, resulting in significant yield reductions. Weeds often take nitrogen and potassium out of the soil. Both in the rhizosphere and the atmosphere, weeds battle for space. Crops achieve a lower photosynthesis when there are weeds because they have less room to grow their shoots. Weeds also damage food crops, which have negative effects on both people and animals when ingested.

Weed detection and control is costly when done manually. Thus deep learning techniques come in handy for weed detection. Being able to accurately detect and identify weeds is a critical initial step in the implementation of an autonomous weed control system. It might be difficult to find weeds in crops. Obstruction (Figure 5.1), color, and texture similarity (Figure 5.2), shadowed plants, the difference in lighting sconditions cause disparity in color and texture, and different species of weeds that look similar are all typical challenges in crop and weed identification and categorization. During different growth periods, identical agricultural plants or weeds may display differences. The challenge of categorizing plants is further made more difficult by motion blur and visual noise. In addition, the types of weeds might differ based on the environment, crop variety, weather, and soil conditions.

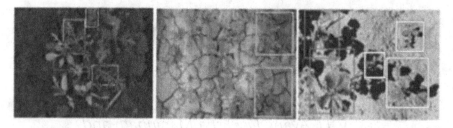

FIGURE 5.1 Common challenges in the identification and classification of crops and weed.

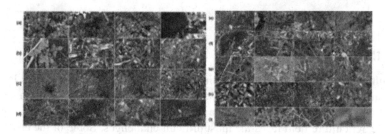

FIGURE 5.2 Specimen images from every weed class (a) Chinee apple, (b) Lantana, (c) Parkinsonia, (d) Parthenium, (e) Prickly acacia, (f) Rubber vine, (g) Siam weed, (h) Snake weed and (i) Negatives [13].

Strong neural networks have an advantage in distinguishing weeds and seedlings when compared to typical human characteristics (such as color, texture, and form), and they can discriminate the background from the identified items to provide the impact of correct recognition. To automatically create a feature extractor and classifier suited for the recognition job, for the extraction of features of the input material, and conduction of a regression estimate, a convolutional neural network is used [26].

This problem of weed management can be solved or overcome by using deep learning techniques [31]. These methods involve intensive feature selection or identification and categorize various types of weeds and also distinguish them from the useful crops cultivated. The weeds that can be identified are as follows: Chinee apple, (2) Lantana, (3) Parkinsonia, (4) Parthenium, (5) Prickly acacia, (6) Rubber vine, (7) Siam weed, (8) Snake weed, (9) others (negatives). Images of every class are shown in Figure 5.2.

The five main phases of a typical classification model of weeds are picture capture, preprocessing, such as image enhancement, feature extraction or feature selection, using an machine learning-based classifier, and performance evaluation. Differentiating between weeds and crops may be done by extracting form characteristics. Color and texture are some further characteristics. From the supplied training data, machine learning techniques learn the features. The training data was acquired from an open data repository called DeepWeeds. This consists of 17,509 unique weed images with nine classes (mentioned above).

Introduction to Disease Prediction

The usage of automated plant-type identification procedures might thus be of considerable assistance to farmers in terms of pesticide and fertilizing and also harvesting to improve the quality of crops. By identifying or detecting the weeds in the fields, farmers can take appropriate measures to control them. Some of the adopted methods include the use of herbicides and fungicides.

To summarize, the development of an autonomous weed detection system has as its main goal the provision of a weed control strategy that will minimize expense and maximize crop yields [29].

5.2 LITERATURE REVIEW

Extensive research is being done in the area of deep learning (DL) in agriculture. DL is employed for the detection of weeds from plants consisting of edible crops and weeds and thereby classification of the weeds detected. To categorize plants in agriculture, machine learning (ML) and deep learning (DL) based approaches such as convolutional neural networks can be used. The usage of automated plant-type identification procedures might thus be of considerable assistance to farmers in terms of pesticide and fertilizing, and also harvesting, which would improve the quality of crops.

In Jacob L. et al.'s research work, a system is developed in which the crop is examined and recognized based on its features, and then the main and minor illnesses are diagnosed using a disease detection approach based on the user's photo. Following the picture segmentation and image preprocessing methods, the neural network classifier is used for that image, and the pests and weeds are detected by pattern and measurement of that pattern [1].

Many current approaches for detecting plants in imagery assume that plant leaves do not overlap, which is frequently broken, lowering the efficiency of the approaches currently used. One of the approaches in M. Dyrmann et al.'s work solves the problem by using a convoluted neural network (CNN) to construct a pixel-by-pixel categorization of the soil, weeds, and crops in red, green, blue (RGB) photos from fields, allowing researchers to determine the location of the plants precisely. The top-down views of weeds and corn in fields that are replicated are used for training. The findings demonstrate pixel precision of 94% [2].

All systems and studies recommend a comprehensive weed control that satisfies a set of essential requirements. Rather than segmenting the image into individual leaves or plants to assess crop or weed confidence at sparse pixel coordinates on the basis of characteristics collected from a wide overlapping neighborhood, a Random Forest classifier is utilized when ultra-high precision weed management is required for specific crops. The average classification accuracy of one suggested method by Florian J. Knoll et al., wherein cross-validation in a leave-one-out scheme is performed on the photos from the dataset, is 93% [3].

S. Jeba Priya et al.'s research involved the segregation of crops and weeds based on their color and physical characteristics. In certain circumstances, the weeds' characteristics are retrieved using the Herpes simplex virus color space technique, which has greater accuracy than the RGB color space model. When compared to the support vector method (SVM) approach [30], for better results, the feature that is extracted is compared to the training data in CNNs. For a more accurate value, a neural network is utilized to split the pictures into pixels. A maximum accuracy of around 95% can be achieved [4].

Some approaches mentioned in Radhika Kamath et al. involve detecting weeds, followed by localization and then classification. Weed mapping for density can be beneficial for weed control since it can lead to less pesticide usage and consequently higher plant quality. For the purpose of mapping the density of weeds in a field, the DL approach has been used in several studies. A map of the field based on the distribution of weeds is constructed using a deep learning method. Farmers may keep track of weed distribution and spread and take action as needed. Semantic segmentation models such as PSPNet, UNet, and SegNet were explored in Radhika Kamath et al.'s research work for segmenting paddy crops along with two varieties of weeds that are found in paddy fields – broadleaved weed and sedges weed. The technique of semantic segmentation is preferred in the case of real-time segmentation of weeds in fields and the models are based on a typical CNN network. Three semantic segmentation models (ResNet-50 was used as the foundation model) were employed for segmenting paddy crops and the two kinds of weeds mentioned: SegNet, Pyramid Scene Parsing Network (PSPNetl), and UNet. This study's findings were compared to traditional ML approaches and segmentation models such as fully convolutional networks. When compared to UNet and SegNet, PSPNet fared better. The result was good, with the mean internal optical urethrotomy (IoU) ranging from 70% to 80% and the frequency-weighted IoU ranging from 80% to 90% [5].

Multi-feature fusion and SVM methods were used in Chen Y et al.'s work. These methods are based on image segmentation using K-mean clustering, considering color information and connected region analysis. Following feature extraction of weeds and seedlings (of corn), the principal component analysis technique was employed to reduce dimensionality. The recognition model was developed with SVM as the classifier. Based on the comparison of a single feature or varied strategies of fusion (for six features), an optimal feature fusion strategy was obtained. An accuracy of around 96% (detected corn seedlings and weeds accurately) was obtained using the SVM classifier [6].

The main objective as proposed by R. Kingsy Grace et al. was to differentiate (or detect) weeds from other edible crops using a DL approach. To categorize the various sorts of weeds and crops, the CNN – VGG16 was utilized. Using filters, features were extracted from images using the convolutional layer. In the hidden layer, the extensively used activation function in CNN, ReLU (Rectified Linear Unit), was employed and softmax was employed in the fully connected layer. The model was developed using Google Colaboratory and gave an accuracy of around 89% [7].

C.T. Selvi et al.'s study proposes a deep learning framework based on image processing to categorize diverse crops and weeds. By extending the deep layers in comparison to the existing CNN, a deep convoluted neural network architecture is built to accomplish this categorization with enhanced accuracy. An image input layer, convolutional two-dimensional layers, rectified linear unit layers, two-dimensional max-pooling layers, fully connected layers, soft-max, and a classification layer are all

Introduction to Disease Prediction

part of the suggested convolutional neural network design. An accuracy of 95% was obtained by utilizing a CNN with max-pooling layers, with a lower rate of weed and crop misclassification [8].

Urmashev et al. used YOLOv5 architecture to create a weed detection system. For the purpose of weed detection, on employing K-nearest neighbors, an accuracy of 83.3% was obtained, Random Forest, an accuracy of 87.5% was obtained and Decision Tree Classifier, an accuracy of 80% was obtained according to the evaluation findings. The primary distinction between YOLO and other object identification CNN methods is that it detects objects in real time very quickly [9].

A. Subeesh et al. investigated the feasibility of DL-based approaches (Alexnet, GoogLeNet, InceptionV3, and Xception) in the detection of weeds from photos (RGB) of a bell pepper field. The selected models' total accuracy ranged from 94.5% to 97.7%. The InceptionV3 model performed the best [10].

5.3 IMPLEMENTATION

5.3.1 BLOCK DIAGRAM

Figure 5.3 depicts a block diagram of the different stages of implementation, each of which are explained in detail below.

5.3.2 DATASET

The dataset used for the implementation of this project is DeepWeeds. This is an open source dataset repository. The dataset consisted of 17,509 distinct color images of nine different classes of weeds. The classes are: (1) Chinee apple, (2) Lantana, (3) Parkinsonia, (4) Parthenium, (5) Prickly acacia, (6) Rubber vine, (7) Siam weed, (8) Snake weed, and (9) others (negatives). The images are of 256×256 resolution. In this dataset, 15,007 images were used for training purposes and 2,501 for validation or testing purposes. These photos were taken on-site in eight different rangeland situations across the globe. Table 5.1 shows the number of images in each aforementioned class.

The dataset was acquired by the following methods. One of the approaches is by using unmanned aerial vehicles. Other than this, various types of field robots are used to compile the images required. Another acquisition method is utilizing all-terrain vehicles with cameras mounted on them. Images can also be collected by satellites. Tensorflow datasets consist of pre-loaded datasets including DeepWeeds.

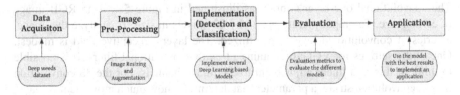

FIGURE 5.3 Block diagram representing end-to-end implementation.

TABLE 5.1
Number of images of each type of weed

Weed	No. of Images	Weed	No. of Images
Chinee apple	1125	Rubber vine	1009
Lantana	1064	Siam weed	1074
Parkinsonia	1031	Snake weed	1016
Part henium	1022	Others (negatives)	9106
Prickly acacia	1062		

Thus, the DeepWeeds dataset can be directly imported into the program using simple TensorFlow snippet code.

5.3.3 Image Loading and Preprocessing

Image preprocessing involves techniques or operations applied to the images in order to make them suitable for training the deep learning model. The images of DeepWeeds are of the size of 256*256*3. The resolution of the color images is resized to 224*224 pixels in order to maintain uniformity. The images were normalized by dividing the image array by 255.

Another preprocessing technique is data augmentation. The same was adopted in order to avoid overfitting and thereby increase the accuracy of the DL model. The augmentation approaches were implemented:

1. Adjusting or rather altering the brightness of the image with a random brightness factor. This ensures the weed images taken under any brightness level are acknowledged.
2. Randomly flipping the image horizontally and vertically. This ensures the weed images taken at any angle are acknowledged.
3. Adjusting the hue and contrast of the image by a random factor.
4. Rotating the image by 90 degrees.

All the aforementioned techniques were implemented using TensorFlow functions.

5.3.4 Deep Learning-Based Models

5.3.4.1 VGG 16 and VGG19

The convolutional one-layer's input, as illustrated in Figure 5.4, is an RGB image of certain size. The input picture is 224 by 224 pixels in size. To analyze the image, a series of convolutional layers are utilized. The layers' receptive field is modest. One of the settings for VGG16 contains 11 extra convolutional filters. It is possible to think of this as a linear adjustment to the input channels. For the 33 convolution layers, convolution stride, a parameter that determines how much movement is made,

Introduction to Disease Prediction

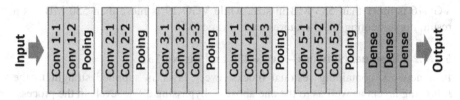

FIGURE 5.4 VGG-16 architecture layout.

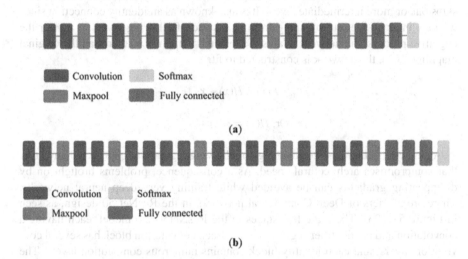

FIGURE 5.5 Schematic representation of VGG16 and VGG19 [14].

is set at 1 pixel. The convolutional layer's input spatial padding is set to the same amount. For the purpose of maintaining spatial resolution, this operation is carried out after convolution. Spatial pooling is a function of the convolutional layers that were followed by the max-pooling layers, which were five in number. The parameter for mobility in an image known as stride is set to 2 enabling max-pooling over a 2 × 2 pixel frame. Convolutional layers are followed by three completely linked layers. The first and second layers each have 4,096 channels, while the third layer does a 1,000-way ILSVRC classification using 1,000 channels (one for each class). It is mostly employed for object identification and picture categorization. The soft-max layer is the final one. The levels that are fully connected in all networks are set up similarly. Well after the 12th convolutional layer, VGG-19 [22] has three more convolutional layers than VGG-16.

All networks, with the exception of one, adopt local response normalization since it increases computation time, increases memory consumption, and does not improve ILSVRC performance. The VGG-based models in Figure 5.5 offer various benefits, such as the fact that pre-trained networks for VGG are easy to build and comprehend, and that it is a particularly ideal architecture for benchmarking on a particular purpose. On the other hand, VGGNet has two drawbacks. One, it moves quite slowly.

VGG16 is more than 533 MB in size, while VGG-19 is more than 550 MB. As a result, implementing VGG requires a lot of time [35].

5.3.4.2 Residual Network – ResNet50 and ResNet152

In a network containing residual blocks, every layer is supplied straight to the following layers as well as to the one above it, bypassing a few levels in the process. With residual blocks, we can train neural networks much more deeply. The link, shown by a curved arrow, is referred to as a forgo connection or bypass connection since it skips one or more intermediate levels. It is also known as an identity connection since we may infer an identity mapping from it. Instead of allowing layers to master the cognitive process, the network adapts the residual mapping. Rather than the original mapping, $H(x)$, the network is constructed to fit,

$$F(x) = H(x) - x$$

$$\text{Or, } H(x) = F(x) + x$$

A skip connection has the advantage of allowing regularization to avoid any layer that compromises architectural speed. As a consequence, problems brought on by disappearing gradients can be avoided while training very deep neural networks. There are 50 tiers of Deep Conv neural networks in the ResNet 50 design, as seen in Figure 5.6 [23]. There are five stages in the ResNet50 2.0 model, each having a convolution and an identifier segment chunk. Each convolution block has several convolution layers, and each identity block contains numerous convolution layers. The ResNet 150 has over 23M parameters that can be trained. According to the aforementioned justification, ResNet is quicker and more accurate than VGG [35].

ResNet152 is less difficult despite the fact it has 152 tiers and also is eight times larger than VGG nets. Rather than processing the data directly, it gains knowledge of the functions expressed in residual form.

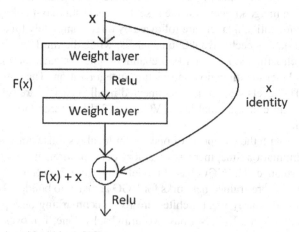

FIGURE 5.6 A residual block [15].

Introduction to Disease Prediction

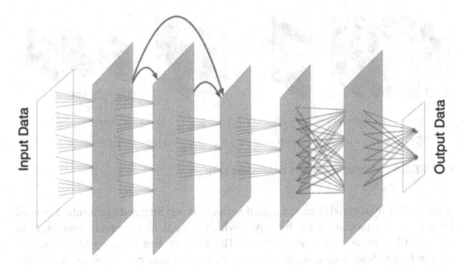

FIGURE 5.7 DenseNet architecture [16].

5.3.4.3 DenseNet121 and DenseNet201

The architecture seen in Figure 5.7 is known as DenseNet because every layer is coupled with every other layer. There are direct links that are (½)*L*(L+1) for L layers. Prior feature maps are regarded as the input for each layer, and the feature maps of that layer are taken into consideration as the input for subsequent layers. The input for a layer in DenseNet is a fusion of feature maps from earlier levels. This results in fewer channels, higher computational, and memory efficiency, as well as a less-bulky network. With extracted feature maps of the quantity of channels, they are employed for every layer where after they are used for 33 convolutional layers [35].

Following are a few benefits of DenseNet versus VGG and ResNet. First, earlier levels may more easily detect errors. Since the top classification layer may provide direct supervision to lower layers, this is a form of implicit deep supervision. The parameters of ResNet are related to channels scaled by the rate of growth for each layer, as opposed to DenseNet's parameters, which are related to channels times the rate of growth for each layer. As a result, DenseNet is much smaller than ResNet. This feature is crucial for simplifying calculation and, as a result, cutting down on execution time.

Thirdly, DenseNet has more variegated features and tends to have patterns because each layer receives all prior layers as input [24]. Finally, the classifier in DenseNet uses characteristics of all degrees of intricacies. It tends to provide more fluid decision-making boundaries. It also explains why even in the limited amount of training data, DenseNet performs effectively [25].

5.3.4.4 MobileNet and MobileNetV2

Figure 5.8 depicts the MobileNet architecture. A complete convolutional layer only exists in the first layer. The additional convolutional layers may all be divided and separated based on their depth. Only the last layer, which has no non-linearity and is completely linked, is unaffected by batch normalizing and ReLU non-linearity. It

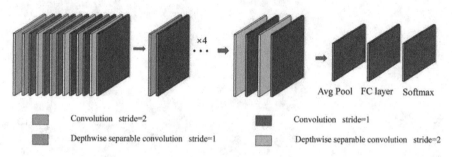

FIGURE 5.8 MobileNet standard architecture [17].

is succeeded by a classification-focused softmax layer. Stripped convolution is used for depthwise convolution, the first layer, which is a complete convolutional layer as discussed before, and for downsampling. The 28 years that make up MobileNet, as seen in Figure 5.8, contain depth wise as well as pointwise convolutional layers that are taken into separate consideration [27].

The following are a few benefits of MobileNet. The first change is a smaller network. Second, there are less parameters now. Thirdly, it performs better and is lighter. MobileNet has a low latency aspect.

With its Depthwise Separable Convolution, MobileNet is perfect for mobile devices or any other devices with constrained processing power since it dramatically decreases the complexity, expense, and dimension of the network. In MobileNetV2, an improved component with an overturned residual structure is shown. Systematic segmentation and object identification execute at a high level thanks to MobileNetV2's support for feature extraction.

5.3.4.5 InceptionNetV3 and InceptionResNetV2

The architecture of InceptionNet excludes a sequential model. Instead, as illustrated in Figure 5.9, the design is such that each convolutional layer's output is supplied to a separate layer concurrently. As a result, the model is trained concurrently, and all outputs are then concatenated. Information loss happens when processes are carried out simultaneously. However, it is perfectly good since if a convolution operation will produce a certain characteristic, another operation will too [28]. The module extracts several characteristics from every convolution or pooling process since each operation draws a certain kind of input or information.

The characteristics collected will be combined with all the acquired data in a single feature map after the concurrent completion of individual features. The model concentrates on numerous aspects at once. As a consequence, accuracy is enhanced. Due to the fact that a distinct kernel size is taken into account for each operation, the output scale of each extracted feature map will differ. The various feature maps that were collected are merged to yield the same output size for all procedures using the padding technique.

InceptionNet has more adaptability and requires less time for training, which are two benefits of this model. This has the disadvantage that bigger InceptionNet models are more likely to overfit, especially when there aren't enough label instances.

Introduction to Disease Prediction

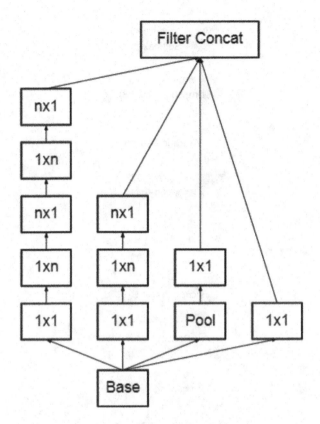

FIGURE 5.9 The fundamental concept used by InceptionNet: The output of one layer is fed to different layers, all of them training in parallel [18].

The 1,064-layer CNN Inception-ResNet-v2 network was trained using more than 1M images from the ImageNet repository. It can group pictures into more than a thousand distinct categories. As a result, the network has acquired knowledge about a variety of feature descriptions for a variety of images. A 299 × 299 image is input to the network, which then outputs a series of inferred class possibilities [35].

The preceding structure is developed using the residual relation and inception structure. Convolutional filters of various sizes are used with residual connections in the Inception–Resnet component. In addition to removing the degradation problem that deep structures create, the usage of residual connections also cuts training time by 50%.

The network's first layers are depicted in Figure 5.10 and consist of three classic layers of convolution, a max-pooling phase, two convolutional layers, and then a max-pooling layer. The following phase of the network contains inception convolution, which requires convolving the input several times with different filter lengths for every convolution, combining the results, and then providing them to the residual network [19].

When the network approaches the termination point, it employs dropout layers to arbitrarily let go of the weights to prevent overfitting. The network then continuously

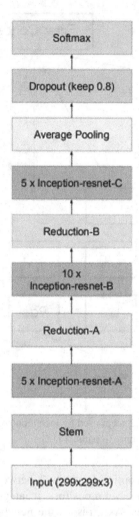

FIGURE 5.10 Architecture of Inception-Resnet-V2 [19].

reruns inceptions as well as residuals, with certain sections repeating 20 or more times. Additionally, the second outer layer is a fully interconnected layer that influences all neurons according to the knowledge acquired. The scores are then probabilistically distributed to the ultimate thousand neurons using softmax [19].

In terms of effectiveness and accuracy, the Inception-ResNet-v2 architecture fares better than earlier sophisticated models.

5.3.5 Proposed Model

Figure 5.11 depicts the complete architecture of the implemented deep learning model. The input image of the type: float32 [1] is fed to the model. A padding

Introduction to Disease Prediction

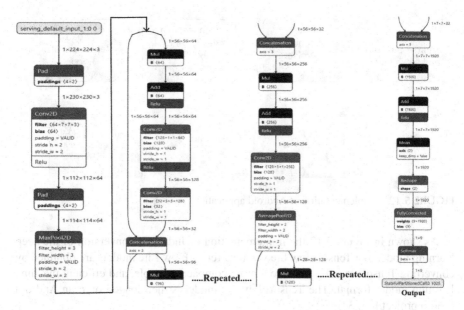

FIGURE 5.11 Architecture of the model which gave the best results.

process is performed to provide filtered images to the convolutional layers. The padded images are given to the convolutional 2D layer with a filter size of (64 × 7 × 7 × 7) and a bias of (64) along with the Relu activation function. The output on which the padding process takes place again is given to a Max-pooling 2D layer. The output obtained after performing this process repeatedly is then flattened (reshaped) and then given to the fully connected layer with weights and biases applied. This process ends with a softmax function wherein the probabilities of the occurrence of all classes are calculated and the output returned is the class with the highest probability [32].

The ReLu layer increases total network speed. Images were down-sampled using max-pooling layers. To flatten the input picture, fully connected layers of neurons of varying sizes are employed. The softmax layer classifies the processed picture [8].

Callbacks have been used in the model for training to avoid overfitting by using EarlyStopping. The optimization function used is Adam, the loss function used is sparse categorical cross entropy and accuracy is the metric used.

5.3.6 ANDROID MOBILE APPLICATION

The application was created using Android Studio and the programming language used was Java. Google's Android Studio is the Android operating system's official integrated development environment. It is based on the IntelliJ IDEA software from JetBrains and is solely used for Android development [12].

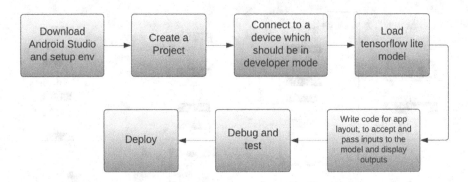

FIGURE 5.12 Implementation of Android application.

As shown in Figure 5.12 the implementation includes the conversion of the deep learning model to a TensorFlow lite version. TensorFlow Lite models are obtained by converting TensorFlow models into a more compact, portable, and efficient machine learning model format. The TensorFlow lite model is then loaded onto an Android Studio project [33, 34].

To run TensorFlow Lite deep learning models, certain project dependencies have to be added to the build.gradle file such as

- TensorFlow Lite main library – The essential data input classes, execution of the model imported, and output obtained after the model is executed are provided by this library.
- TensorFlow Lite Support library – To convert or translate the uploaded images into a TensorImage data object that can be processed by the imported ML model, this library provides a helper class.
- TensorFlow Lite GPU library – Support is provided by this library to accelerate the ML model execution using GPU processors on the device, if available.

Utility functions have to be included in the code to convert data to a tensor data format that can be processed by the imported model. The image uploaded by the user is converted to float32 [1, 224, 224, 3] format. Each pixel of the image is iterated over and the extracted R, G, and B values are added to a buffer. This buffer is provided as input to the model for prediction. The outputs obtained from the model are in the form of a Tensor buffer, which is then converted to an array of data type "float" for further processes. The array is analyzed and the weed label with the highest confidence is returned.

Figure 5.13 shows the design of the application. The launch gallery button, when clicked by the user, will request the user to select the gallery of his/her choice. The image uploaded by the user appears in the ImageView space and the classification output appears in the space below the image following the text "Classified as:"

The application is designed such that it is very simple to use. As shown in Figure 5.14 the user is only required to upload an image following which the output will be displayed in the app.

Introduction to Disease Prediction

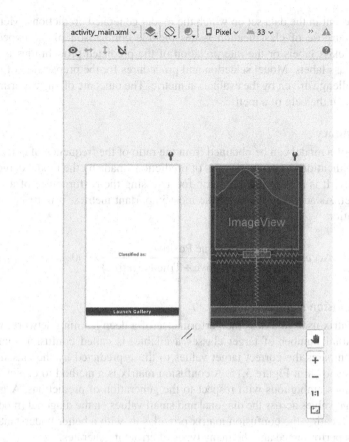

FIGURE 5.13 App layout on Android Studio.

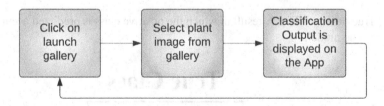

FIGURE 5.14 Steps to use the application.

5.4 EVALUATION

5.4.1 Evaluation Metrics

Evaluation metrics quantify a prediction model's capabilities. Typically, it requires training of a model on a data set, following which predictions are generated by the model on a data set (not used before). The predictions are then compared to the values (predicted) present in the data set on which the model generated predictions. Metrics used for the purpose of classification issues include comparison of the expected and predicted class labels or the interpretation of the predicted probabilities of the problem for class labels. Model selection and procedures for the preparation of data is a search challenge driven by the evaluation metric. The outcome of any experiment is quantified with the help of a metric.

5.4.1.1 Accuracy

The accuracy of a model can be obtained from the ratio of the frequency of correctly predicted classifications to the total count of predictions made by the model depicted in Equation 5.1. It is a quantifiable metric for assessing the performance of a deep learning model. As accuracy is one of the most important metrics, it must be taken into consideration.

$$\text{Accuracy} = \frac{\text{True Positive}}{(\text{True Positive} + \text{True Negative})} \times 100 \qquad (5.4.1)$$

5.4.1.2 Confusion Matrix

An N-by-N matrix used to assess the performance of a deep learning network, with N being the total number of target classes available, is called confusion matrix. The matrix compares the correct target values to those predicted by the classification model, as shown in Figure 5.15. A confusion matrix is a method to depict how a model becomes ambiguous with respect to the generation of predictions. A good matrix has large values across the diagonal and small values on the diagonal (model). Measuring or locating the confusion matrix provides us with a better understanding of the model's performance and the many types of errors it generates.

Components of a Confusion Matrix:

1. True positive (TP): A result in which the positive class is predicted accurately by the model.

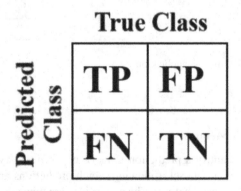

FIGURE 5.15 Confusion matrix for binary classification.

Introduction to Disease Prediction

2. False negative (FN): A result where the negative class is predicted wrongly by the model.
3. False positive (FP): A result where the positive class is predicted wrongly by the model.
4. True negative (TN): A result where the negative class is predicted accurately by the model.

Confusion Matrix for Multi-label Classification:
Figure 5.16 represents the confusion matrix of a three-class classification issue. To explain how a confusion matrix works for a multi-class classification issue, three classes (A, B, and C) have been studied.

TP_A, TP_B, and TP_C are the true positive (TP) values of the classes A, B and C respectively.

Consider class A. E_{AB} and E_{AC} are the samples from class A that were misclassified as B and C, respectively, and are referred to as misclassified samples. The class A false negative (FN), FN_A, is the total of all class A samples that were incorrectly categorized as class B or class C.

$$FN_A = E_{AB} + E_{AC} \qquad (5.2)$$

Consider class A. E_{BA} represents the samples from class B misclassified as class A and E_{CA} represents the samples from class C misclassified as class A. False positive (FP) of class A (Equation 5.3) is obtained by finding the sum of all the incorrectly classified samples in the first row:

$$FP_A = E_{BA} + E_{CA} \qquad (5.3)$$

The false negative of any class (Equations 5.4–5.7) is found by adding the incorrectly classified samples in that column and a FP for any predicted class can be found by adding the incorrectly classified samples in that row [11].

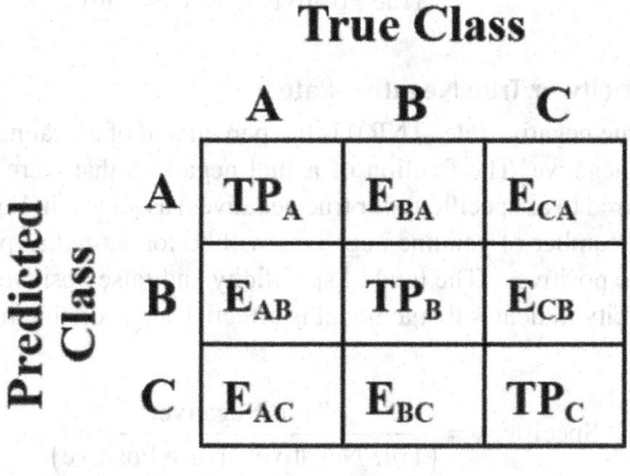

		True Class		
Predicted Class		A	B	C
	A	TP_A	E_{BA}	E_{CA}
	B	E_{AB}	TP_B	E_{CB}
	C	E_{AC}	E_{BC}	TP_C

FIGURE 5.16 Confusion matrix for multi-label classification.

$$FN_B = E_{BA} + E_{BC} \quad (5.4)$$

$$FP_B = E_{AB} + E_{CB} \quad (5.5)$$

$$FN_C = E_{CA} + E_{CB} \quad (5.6)$$

$$FP_C = E_{AC} + E_{BC} \quad (5.7)$$

True negative (TN) values of a class (Equations 5.8–5.10) are found by adding all samples in all the rows and columns except the row and column containing the class for which the true negative value is being calculated.

$$TN_A = TP_A + E_{CB} + E_{BC} + TP_C \quad (5.8)$$

$$TN_B = TP_A + E_{CA} + E_{AC} + TP_C \quad (5.9)$$

$$TN_C = TP_A + E_{BA} + E_{AB} + TP_B \quad (5.10)$$

Considering an m x m confusion matrix,

$$\text{Number of correct classifications that are possible} = m \quad (5.11)$$

$$\text{Number of errors possible} = m^2 - m \quad (5.12)$$

5.4.1.3 Sensitivity or Recall or False Positive Rate

Sensitivity is defined as the proportion of TP to actual positives in the data, as shown in Equation 5.13. Sensitivity refers to a test's capability to accurately identify a weed.

A model that has a high value of sensitivity will have fewer false negatives. For the detection of weeds, sensitivity of a model is a crucial factor.

$$\text{Sensitivity} = \frac{\text{True Positive}}{(\text{True Positive} + \text{False Negative})} \quad (5.13)$$

5.4.1.4 Specificity or True Negative Rate

Specificity (or true negative rate (TNR)) is the percentage of actual negatives that are projected to be negative. The fraction of actual negatives that were expected to be negatives is referred to as specificity (or true negatives) as shown in Equation 5.14. As a result, a small number of genuine negatives will be forecasted as positives (sometimes called false positives). The total of specificity and false positive rates is always 1. A high specificity indicates that a model is effective at predicting true negatives.

$$\text{Specificity} = \frac{\text{True Negative}}{(\text{True Negative} + \text{False Positive})} \quad (5.14)$$

Introduction to Disease Prediction

5.4.1.5 Precision

Precision is defined as the fraction of positive data points accurately categorized to total positive data points correctly or wrongly categorized as depicted in Equation 5.15. Precision decreases when the deep learning model generates a limited number of positive classifications or several incorrect accurate (positive) classifications. Whereas the precision increases when a few incorrect positive classifications or multiple correct positive classifications are made by the classification model developed.

$$\text{Precision} = \frac{\text{True Positive}}{(\text{True Positive} + \text{False Positive})} \quad (5.15)$$

5.4.1.6 F1 Score

The mean used between precision and recall is harmonic in the case of F1 score calculation (as shown in Equation 5.16). It is primarily utilized to assess the performance of a DL model. F1 score is utilized when false positives and negatives are significant. One approach to addressing class imbalance concerns is to use better metrics in terms of accuracy, such as F1 score, which takes into account not just the quantity of prediction errors produced by the model, but also the type of errors made.

$$\text{F1 score} = \frac{\text{True Positive}}{\text{True Positive} + 0.5\,(\text{False Positive} + \text{False Negative})} \quad (5.16)$$

5.4.1.7 Negative Predictive Value (NPV)

The proportion of projected negatives that are true negatives is denoted as the negative predictive value (Equation 5.17). It indicates the probability that a projected negative is actually a true negative.

$$\text{NPV} = \frac{\text{True Negative}}{(\text{True Negative} + \text{False Negative})} \quad (5.17)$$

5.4.1.8 False Positive Rate (FPR)

The false-positive rate given by Equation 5.18 is determined by the number of false negatives predicted inaccurately by the model. True positive rate or recall complement FPR. The FPR is best stated as the probability of erroneously rejecting the null hypothesis, which is an important concept in the agricultural area. FPR is one of the measures used to analyze how well ML models perform when used for classification. The lower the incidence of false positives, the better the DL model.

$$\text{FPR} = \frac{\text{False Positive}}{\text{Total no. of Negatives}} = \frac{\text{False Positive}}{(\text{False Positive} + \text{True Negative})} \quad (5.18)$$

5.4.1.9 False Negative Rate (FNR)

FNR, as shown in Equation 5.19, is the proportion of false negatives compared to all negative predictions. True negative rate (TNR) complements FNR. The lower the incidence of false negatives, the better the DL model.

$$\text{FNR} = \frac{\text{False Negative}}{\text{Total no. of Positives}} = \frac{\text{False Negative}}{(\text{False Negative} + \text{True Positive})} \quad (5.19)$$

5.4.1.10 False Discovery Rate (FDR)

FDR is the (predicted) percentage of false-positives among all the significant variables. FDR is the proportion of hypotheses that are wrongly considered to be true (Equation 5.20). 'Discovery' is a test that satisfies the acceptability requirements based on a threshold. FDR is beneficial since it assesses how enriched accepted discoveries are in comparison to actual discoveries.

$$\text{FDR} = \frac{\text{False Positive}}{(\text{False Positive} + \text{True Negative})} \quad (5.20)$$

5.4.1.11 Support, Macro Average and Weighted Average

Support of a class refers to the number of images that belong to that class in the dataset. The number of test images considered for evaluation is 3,502. Hence, support for all the classes is 3,502. The support of "Chinee Apple" is 234 signifying that the number of "Chinee Apple" images in the test dataset is 234. Similarly, support for negatives is 1,771 signifying that the number of images that do not belong to any of the eight weeds classes – Chinee apple, Lantana, Parkinsonia, Parthenium, Prickly acacia, Rubber vine, Siam weed, and Snake weed is 1,771.

The macro-average precision and recall score is generated as an arithmetic means of the precision and recall scores of different classes. The macro average F1 score is derived by taking the arithmetic mean of the F1 scores of all the classes (the F1 score of each class is considered). All the classes are treated equally irrespective of the support values of using this technique. Macro averaging is mostly used to assess the classifier's performance in relation to the most common class labels.

Weighted average considers support when calculating the average of the metrics. If a class has lower support, then the contribution of its precision or recall or F1 score to the weighted average would be lesser. Weighted average is used when the dataset is unbalanced as it considers the support values in its calculations. The contribution of each class to the weighted average is proportional to the support of each class.

$$\text{Macro avg of Precision} = \frac{\text{Prec}_1 + \text{Prec}_2 + \text{Prec}_3 + \ldots + \text{Prec}_n}{n} \quad (5.21)$$

The macro average of Recall and F1 score is calculated similarly (as shown in Equation 5.21):

Introduction to Disease Prediction

Weighted average Calculation:

$$\text{Proportion of a class A} = \frac{\text{Number of samples of class A in the test dataset}}{\text{Total number of samples in the dataset}}$$
$$= \frac{\text{Support of class A}}{\text{Support of all classes}} \qquad (5.22)$$

$$\text{Weighted average of precision} = \text{Prec}_1 * \text{Prop}_1 + \text{Prec}_2 * \text{Prop}_2 + \ldots + \text{Prec}_n * \text{Prop}_n \qquad (5.23)$$

Similarly, for recall and F1 score as well, the weighted average is calculated.

5.5 RESULTS

5.5.1 COMPARISON OF EVALUATION METRICS OF DIFFERENT MODELS

The following results are obtained on training the models for 50 epochs. Support or the number of samples of each label in the test dataset – Chinee apple: 234, Lantana: 211, Parkinsonia: 213, Parthenium: 203, Prickly acacia: 217, Rubber vine: 200, Siam weed: 218, Snake weed: 235, Negatives (any image not belonging to the eight classes of weeds): 1771. Total support or total number of samples in the test dataset: 3,502.

Out of all the models as shown in Table 5.2, the model that gave the best accuracy of 97% and F1 score of 0.97 is DenseNet121.

The loss function may provide more supervision to individual layers via shorter connections, which might explain the higher accuracy of dense convolutional networks. DenseNets are used for "deep supervision." Classifiers are added to each hidden layer in deeply supervised nets, enabling the intermediate layers to acquire discriminative features. Deep supervision is performed implicitly in DenseNets, with

TABLE 5.2
Accuracy obtained for different models

	Deep Learning Model	Overall Accuracy	Weighted Average F1 score
1.	MobileNet	92.55	0.92
2.	MobileNetV2	92.38	0.92
3.	DenseNet121	97.06	0.97
4.	DenseNet201	96.4	0.95
5.	VGG16	94.32	0.94
6.	VGG19	90.23	0.9
7.	InceptionV3	93.4	0.92
8.	InceptionResnetV2	93.77	0.93
9.	Resnet50	94.15	0.93
10.	Resnet152	95.17	0.94

a single classifier on top of the network giving direct supervision to all levels via at most two or three transition layers [20].

Tables 5.3–5.12 provide information about the evaluation metrics obtained for all the classes of weeds for each model used respectively.

5.5.2 Confusion Matrix of Different Deep Learning Models

The threshold considered is the maximum value divided by 2.

The confusion matrices obtained for different models are shown in Figures 5.17–5.26.

5.5.3 Normalized Confusion Matrix of Different Deep Learning Models

The confusion matrix is normalized by dividing the values of a row by the sum of the values of the entire row. The threshold considered is the maximum value divided by 1.5.

The normalized confusion matrices obtained for different models are shown in Figures 5.27–5.36.

5.5.4 Comparative Study of Results Obtained from All the Models Implemented

5.5.4.1 F1 Score

The plots of F1 scores of different weed classes obtained for different models are shown in Figures 5.37–5.44.

5.5.4.2 Recall or Sensitivity

The plots of sensitivity of different weed classes obtained for different models are shown in Figures 5.45–5.52.

5.5.4.3 Precision

The plots of precision of different weed classes obtained for different models are shown in Figures 5.53–5.60.

From the above graphs, it can be observed that for most of the classes of weeds, the highest value of F1 score, recall and sensitivity is obtained when DenseNet121 is used.

5.5.5 Android Mobile Application

The results of the implemented Android mobile application are shown below. Figure 5.61 depicts the basic layout of the mobile application, where the user uploads the intended input image.

Figures 5.62–5.70 represent the output obtained by the mobile application for different classes of weed.

TABLE 5.3
Evaluation metrics for all classes of weeds using MobileNet

	F1 Score	Sensitivity	Specificity	Precision	NPV	FPR	FNR	FDR	Accuracy
Chinee apple	0.78	0.68	0.99	0.91	0.98	0.005	0.32	0.09	0.974
Lantana	0.89	0.91	0.99	0.87	0.99	0.009	0.09	0.13	0.986
Parkinsonia	0.91	0.85	0.99	0.98	0.99	0.001	0.15	0.02	0.99
Parthenium	0.94	0.95	0.99	0.93	0.99	0.004	0.05	0.07	0.993
Prickly acacia	0.90	0.89	0.99	0.91	0.99	0.006	0.11	0.09	0.988
Rubber vine	0.93	0.94	0.99	0.93	0.99	0.004	0.07	0.07	0.992
Siam weed	0.95	0.95	0.99	0.96	0.99	0.003	0.05	0.04	0.994
Snake weed	0.84	0.84	0.99	0.83	0.99	0.012	0.16	0.17	0.978
Negatives	0.95	0.97	0.92	0.93	0.96	0.077	0.03	0.07	0.945

TABLE 5.4
Evaluation metrics for all classes of weeds using MobileNetV2

	F1 Score	Sensitivity	Specificity	Precision	NPV	FPR	FNR	FDR	Accuracy
Chinee apple	0.82	0.78	0.99	0.87	0.98	0.01	0.22	0.13	0.977
Lantana	0.92	0.88	0.99	0.95	0.99	0.002	0.12	0.05	0.99
Parkinsonia	0.92	0.94	0.99	0.89	0.99	0.007	0.06	0.11	0.989
Parthenium	0.88	0.94	0.99	0.82	0.99	0.012	0.06	0.18	0.985
Prickly acacia	0.84	0.98	0.98	0.74	0.99	0.023	0.02	0.26	0.977
Rubber vine	0.92	0.86	0.99	0.98	0.99	0.001	0.14	0.02	0.991
Siam weed	0.94	0.92	0.99	0.97	0.99	0.002	0.08	0.03	0.993
Snake weed	0.87	0.85	0.99	0.88	0.99	0.008	0.15	0.12	0.983
Negatives	0.94	0.94	0.95	0.95	0.94	0.049	0.06	0.05	0.9443

TABLE 5.5
Evaluation metrics for all classes of weeds using DenseNet121

	F1 Score	Sensitivity	Specificity	Precision	NPV	FPR	FNR	FDR	Accuracy
Chinee apple	0.92	0.89	0.99	0.96	0.99	0.002	0.11	0.04	0.99
Lantana	0.97	0.97	0.99	0.96	0.99	0.003	0.33	0.04	0.995
Parkinsonia	0.98	0.99	0.99	0.98	0.99	0.002	0.01	0.02	0.998
Parthenium	0.98	0.96	0.99	0.98	0.99	0.001	0.04	0.02	0.996
Prickly acacia	0.94	0.95	0.99	0.93	0.99	0.005	0.05	0.07	0.992
Rubber vine	0.97	0.96	0.99	0.98	0.99	0.001	0.04	0.02	0.997
Siam weed	0.97	0.95	0.99	0.97	0.99	0.002	0.05	0.03	0.995
Snake weed	0.93	0.91	0.99	0.95	0.99	0.004	0.09	0.05	0.99
Negatives	0.98	0.98	0.97	0.97	0.98	0.034	0.02	0.03	0.975

TABLE 5.6
Evaluation metrics for all classes of weeds using DenseNet201

	F1 Score	Sensitivity	Specificity	Precision	NPV	FPR	FNR	FDR	Accuracy
Chinee apple	0.90	0.87	0.99	0.94	0.99	0.004	0.13	0.06	0.987
Lantana	0.95	0.94	0.99	0.95	0.99	0.003	0.57	0.05	0.993
Parkinsonia	0.95	0.93	0.99	0.97	0.99	0.002	0.66	0.03	0.994
Parthenium	0.97	0.97	0.99	0.98	0.99	0.002	0.23	0.02	0.996
Prickly acacia	0.92	0.95	0.99	0.88	0.99	0.008	0.05	0.12	0.989
Rubber vine	0.96	0.94	0.99	0.97	0.99	0.002	0.06	0.03	0.995
Siam Weed	0.96	0.94	0.99	0.98	0.99	0.002	0.06	0.02	0.995
Snake weed	0.90	0.89	0.99	0.92	0.99	0.006	0.11	0.08	0.987
Negatives	0.97	0.98	0.96	0.96	0.97	0.042	0.02	0.04	0.967

TABLE 5.7
Evaluation metrics for all classes of weeds using VGG16

	F1 Score	Sensitivity	Specificity	Precision	NPV	FPR	FNR	FDR	Accuracy
Chinee apple	0.86	0.81	0.99	0.91	0.99	0.006	0.19	0.09	0.982
Lantana	0.95	0.97	0.99	0.94	0.99	0.004	0.03	0.06	0.994
Parkinsonia	0.97	0.97	0.99	0.97	0.99	0.002	0.03	0.03	0.996
Parthenium	0.94	0.93	0.99	0.95	0.99	0.003	0.07	0.05	0.993
Prickly acacia	0.91	0.94	0.99	0.88	0.99	0.009	0.06	0.12	0.988
Rubber vine	0.96	0.93	0.99	0.99	0.99	0.001	0.08	0.01	0.995
Siam weed	0.96	0.96	0.99	0.96	0.99	0.003	0.04	0.04	0.995
Snake weed	0.88	0.87	0.99	0.90	0.99	0.007	0.13	0.1	0.85
Negatives	0.96	0.97	0.95	0.95	0.97	0.049	0.03	0.05	0.961

TABLE 5.8
Evaluation metrics for all classes of weeds using VGG19

	F1 Score	Sensitivity	Specificity	Precision	NPV	FPR	FNR	FDR	Accuracy
Chinee apple	0.76	0.65	0.99	0.92	0.98	0.004	0.35	0.08	0.973
Lantana	0.87	0.80	0.99	0.95	0.99	0.002	0.2	0.05	0.985
Parkinsonia	0.95	0.95	0.99	0.95	0.99	0.003	0.05	0.05	0.994
Parthenium	0.90	0.91	0.99	0.88	0.99	0.007	0.09	0.12	0.988
Prickly acacia	0.89	0.85	0.99	0.93	0.99	0.004	0.15	0.07	0.987
Rubber vine	0.94	0.94	0.99	0.94	0.99	0.003	0.06	0.06	0.993
Siam weed	0.85	0.98	0.98	0.75	0.99	0.022	0.02	0.25	0.978
Snake weed	0.79	0.83	0.98	0.75	0.99	0.02	0.17	0.25	0.97
Negatives	0.94	0.95	0.93	0.93	0.95	0.068	0.05	0.07	0.94

TABLE 5.9
Evaluation metrics for all classes of weeds using InceptionV3

	F1 Score	Sensitivity	Specificity	Precision	NPV	FPR	FNR	FDR	Accuracy
Chinee apple	0.80	0.71	0.99	0.92	0.98	0.005	0.28	0.08	0.977
Lantana	0.9	0.87	0.99	0.93	0.99	0.004	0.13	0.07	0.988
Parkinsonia	0.94	0.96	0.99	0.91	0.99	0.006	0.04	0.09	0.992
Parthenium	0.92	0.9	0.99	0.94	0.99	0.004	0.09	0.06	0.991
Prickly acacia	0.92	0.94	0.99	0.89	0.99	0.007	0.06	0.11	0.989
Rubber vine	0.91	0.92	0.99	0.9	0.99	0.006	0.08	0.09	0.989
Siam weed	0.93	0.92	0.99	0.94	0.99	0.004	0.08	0.06	0.991
Snake weed	0.86	0.86	0.99	0.86	0.99	0.01	0.14	0.14	0.981
Negatives	0.95	0.96	0.93	0.93	0.96	0.071	0.04	0.07	0.945

TABLE 5.10
Evaluation metrics for all classes of weeds using InceptionResnetV2

	F1 score	Sensitivity	Specificity	Precision	NPV	FPR	FNR	FDR	Accuracy
Chinee apple	0.84	0.79	0.99	0.89	0.99	0.007	0.21	0.11	0.979
Lantana	0.9	0.89	0.99	0.92	0.99	0.005	0.11	0.08	0.989
Parkinsonia	0.94	0.92	0.99	0.95	0.99	0.003	0.08	0.05	0.992
Parthenium	0.93	0.94	0.99	0.92	0.99	0.005	0.06	0.08	0.991
Prickly acacia	0.93	0.94	0.99	0.91	0.99	0.006	0.06	0.09	0.991
Rubber vine	0.93	0.92	0.99	0.94	0.99	0.004	0.09	0.06	0.992
Siam weed	0.96	0.94	0.99	0.98	0.99	0.001	0.06	0.02	0.995
Snake weed	0.86	0.86	0.99	0.86	0.99	0.01	0.14	0.14	0.981
Negatives	0.96	0.97	0.94	0.95	0.97	0.057	0.03	0.05	0.956

TABLE 5.11
Evaluation metrics for all classes of weeds using Resnet50

	F1 score	Sensitivity	Specificity	Precision	NPV	FPR	FNR	FDR	Accuracy
Chinee apple	0.86	0.81	0.99	0.93	0.99	0.004	0.19	0.07	0.983
Lantana	0.94	0.95	0.99	0.94	0.99	0.004	0.05	0.06	0.993
Parkinsonia	0.96	0.99	0.99	0.94	0.99	0.004	0.01	0.06	0.995
Parthenium	0.95	0.96	0.99	0.94	0.99	0.004	0.04	0.06	0.994
Prickly acacia	0.94	0.97	0.99	0.91	0.99	0.006	0.03	0.09	0.992
Rubber vine	0.94	0.94	0.99	0.94	0.99	0.003	0.07	0.06	0.993
Siam weed	0.96	0.96	0.99	0.95	0.99	0.003	0.04	0.05	0.995
Snake weed	0.86	0.88	0.99	0.85	0.99	0.011	0.12	0.15	0.981
Negatives	0.96	0.96	0.97	0.97	0.96	0.034	0.04	0.03	0.965

TABLE 5.12
Evaluation metrics for all classes of weeds using Resnet152

	F1 score	Sensitivity	Specificity	Precision	NPV	FPR	FNR	FDR	Accuracy
Chinee apple	0.87	0.84	0.99	0.9	0.99	0.006	0.16	0.09	0.983
Lantana	0.94	0.96	0.99	0.92	0.99	0.005	0.04	0.08	0.992
Parkinsonia	0.95	0.96	0.99	0.94	0.99	0.004	0.04	0.06	0.994
Parthenium	0.96	0.95	0.99	0.96	0.99	0.002	0.05	0.04	0.995
Prickly acacia	0.95	0.96	0.99	0.94	0.99	0.004	0.04	0.06	0.994
Rubber vine	0.94	0.9	0.99	0.99	0.99	0.003	0.1	0.01	0.994
Siam Weed	0.94	0.91	0.99	0.98	0.99	0.002	0.09	0.02	0.993
Snake Weed	0.87	0.83	0.99	0.92	0.99	0.005	0.17	0.08	0.984
Negatives	0.96	0.98	0.94	0.95	0.98	0.057	0.02	0.05	0.96

Introduction to Disease Prediction

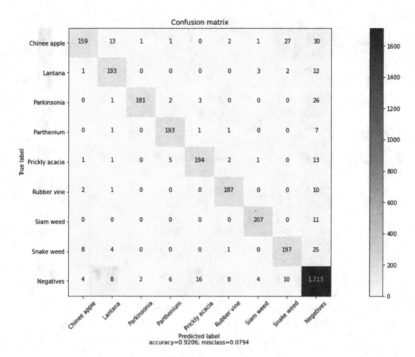

FIGURE 5.17 Confusion matrix of MobileNet.

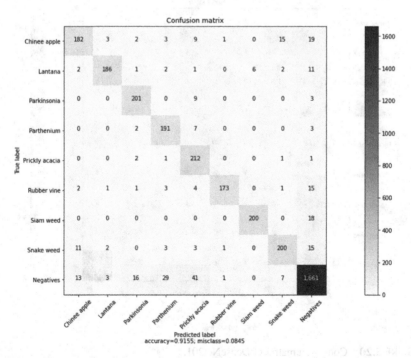

FIGURE 5.18 Confusion matrix of MobileNetV2.

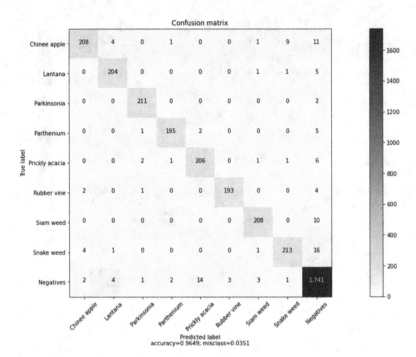

FIGURE 5.19 Confusion matrix of DenseNet121.

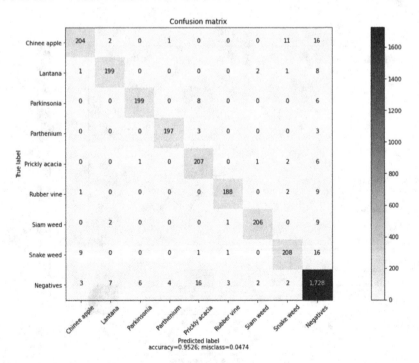

FIGURE 5.20 Confusion matrix of DenseNet201.

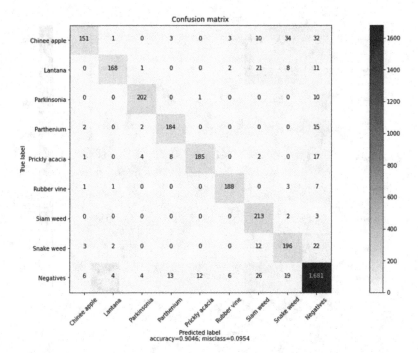

FIGURE 5.21 Confusion matrix of VGG19.

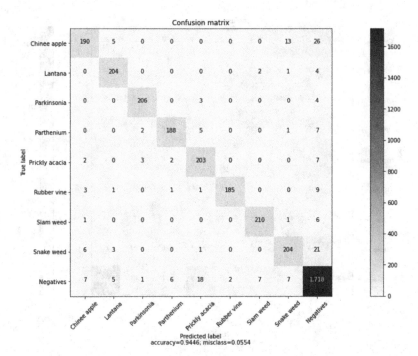

FIGURE 5.22 Confusion matrix of VGG16.

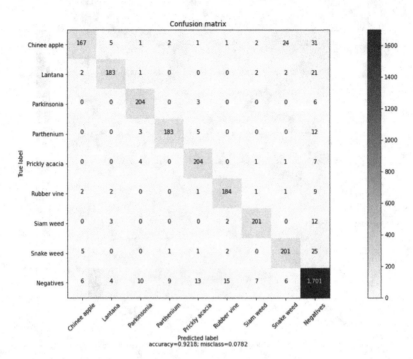

FIGURE 5.23 Confusion matrix of InceptionV3.

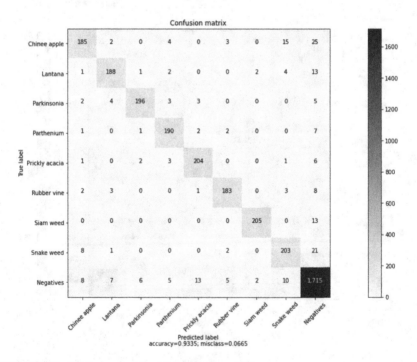

FIGURE 5.24 Confusion matrix of InceptionResnetV2.

Introduction to Disease Prediction

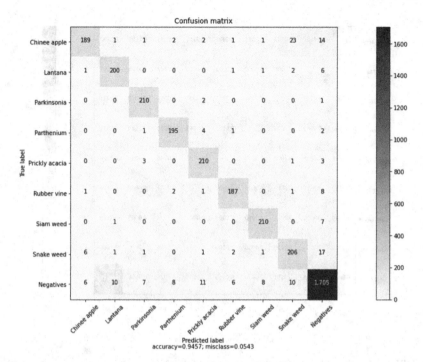

FIGURE 5.25 Confusion matrix of Resnet50.

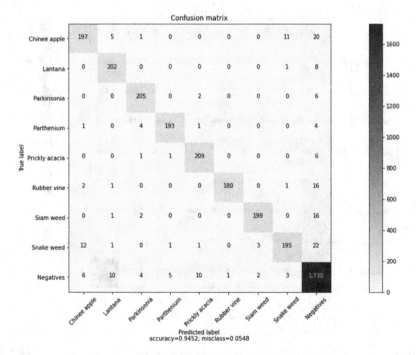

FIGURE 5.26 Confusion matrix of Resnet152.

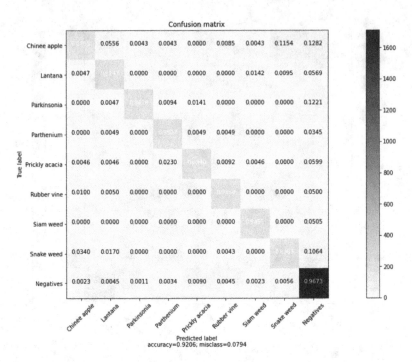

FIGURE 5.27 Normalized confusion matrix of MobileNet.

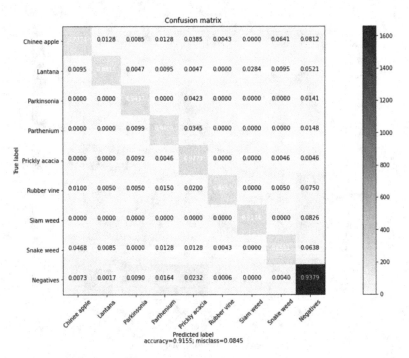

FIGURE 5.28 Normalized confusion matrix of MobileNetV2.

Introduction to Disease Prediction

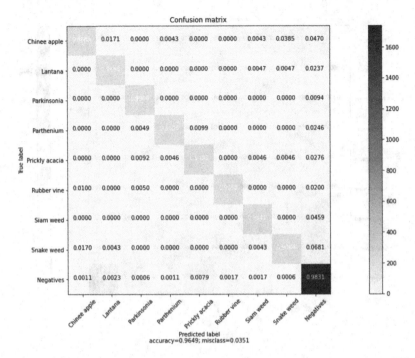

FIGURE 5.29 Normalized confusion matrix of DenseNet121.

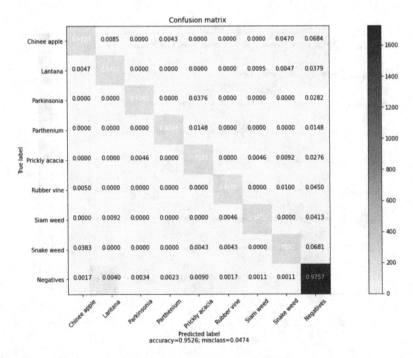

FIGURE 5.30 Normalized confusion matrix of DenseNet201.

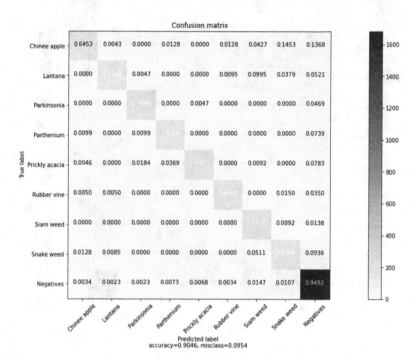

FIGURE 5.31 Normalized confusion matrix of VGG19.

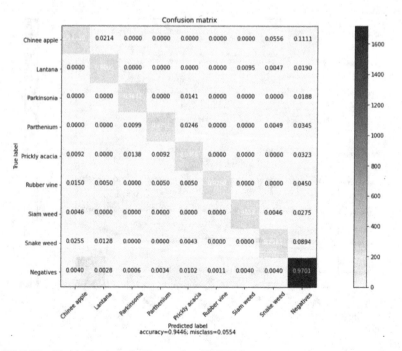

FIGURE 5.32 Normalized confusion matrix of VGG16.

Introduction to Disease Prediction

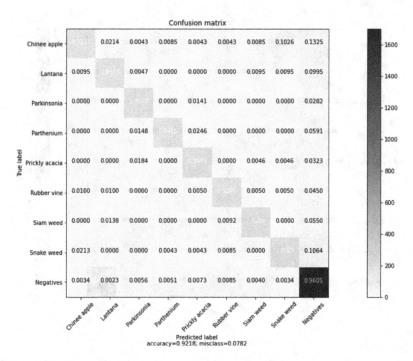

FIGURE 5.33 Normalized confusion matrix of InceptionV3.

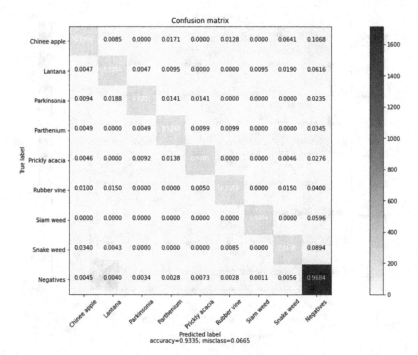

FIGURE 5.34 Normalized confusion matrix of InceptionResnetV2.

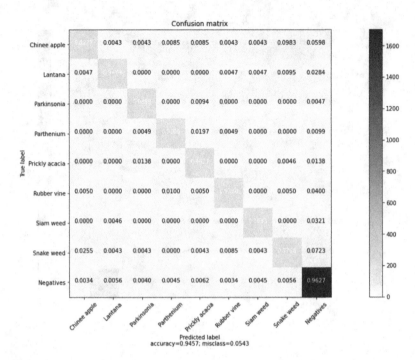

FIGURE 5.35 Normalized confusion matrix of Resnet50.

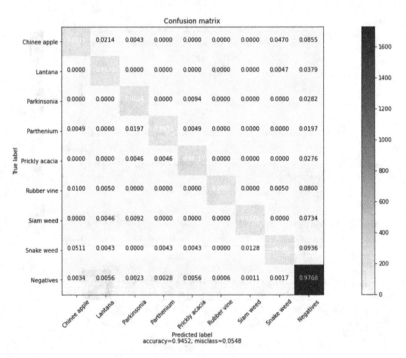

FIGURE 5.36 Normalized confusion matrix of Resnet152.

Introduction to Disease Prediction

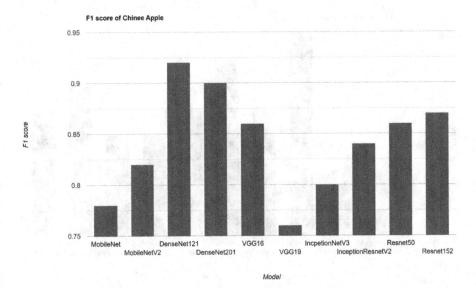

FIGURE 5.37 F1 score of Chinee apple obtained for different models.

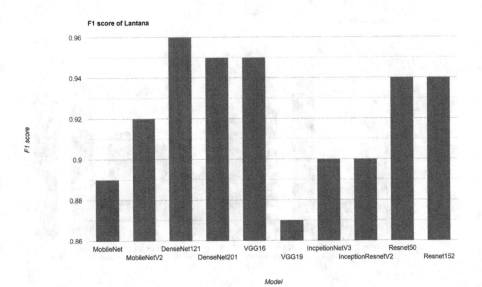

FIGURE 5.38 F1 score of Lantana obtained for different models.

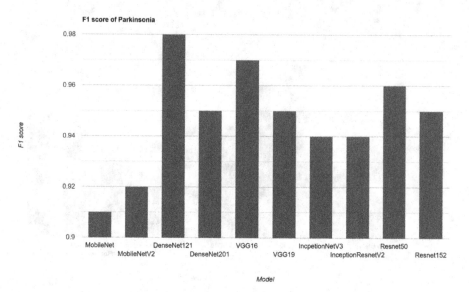

FIGURE 5.39 F1 score of Parkinsonia obtained for different models.

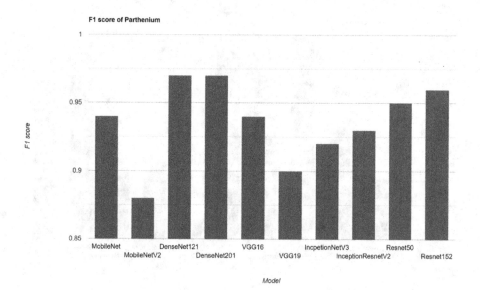

FIGURE 5.40 F1 score of Parthenium obtained for different models.

Introduction to Disease Prediction

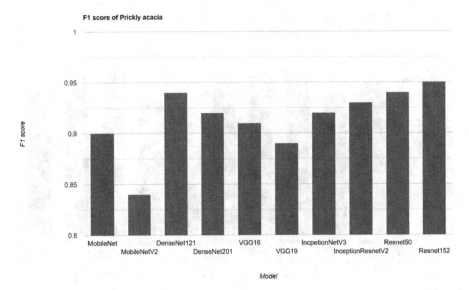

FIGURE 5.41 F1 score of Prickly acacia obtained for different models.

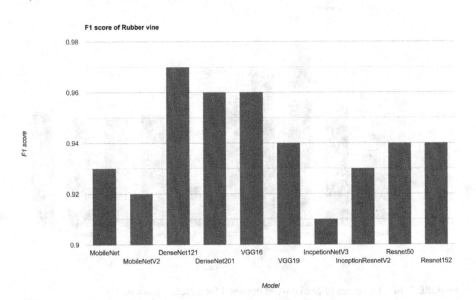

FIGURE 5.42 F1 score of Rubber vine obtained for different models.

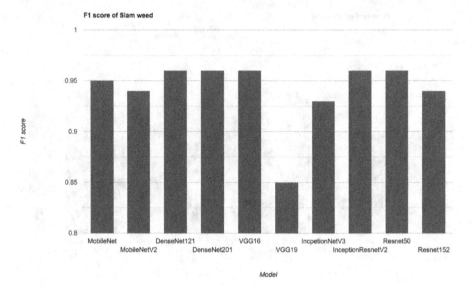

FIGURE 5.43 F1 score of Siam weed obtained for different models.

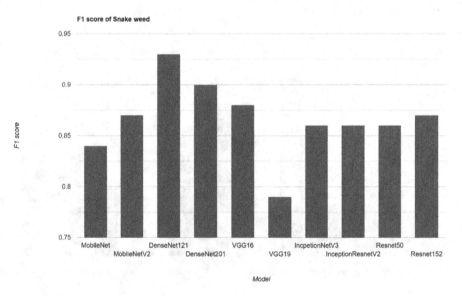

FIGURE 5.44 F1 scores of Snake weed obtained for different models.

Introduction to Disease Prediction

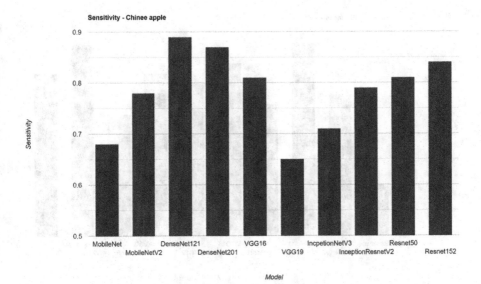

FIGURE 5.45 Sensitivity of Chinee apple obtained for different models.

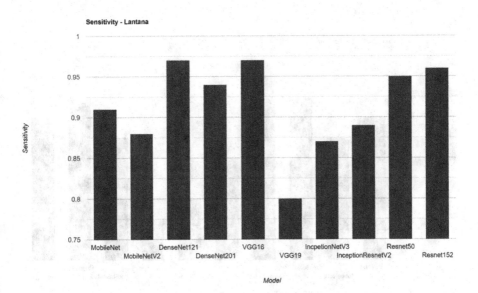

FIGURE 5.46 Sensitivity of Lantana obtained for different models.

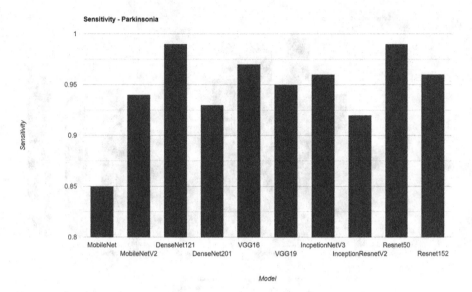

FIGURE 5.47 Sensitivity of Parkinsonia obtained for different models.

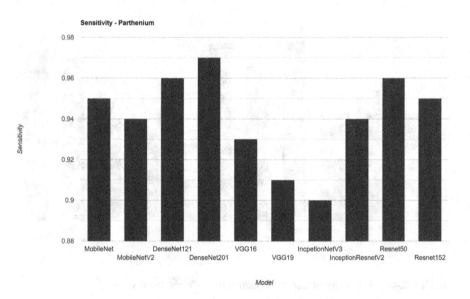

FIGURE 5.48 Sensitivity of Parthenium obtained for different models.

Introduction to Disease Prediction

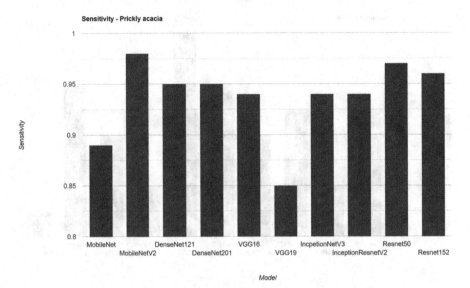

FIGURE 5.49 Sensitivity of Prickly acacia obtained for different models.

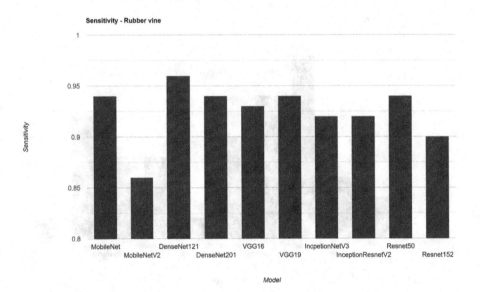

FIGURE 5.50 Sensitivity of Rubber vine obtained for different models.

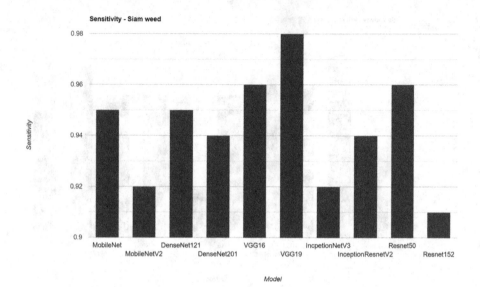

FIGURE 5.51 Sensitivity of Siam weed obtained for different models.

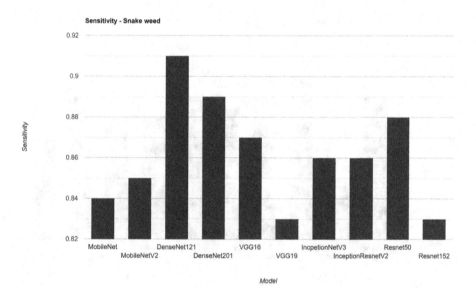

FIGURE 5.52 Sensitivity of Snake weed obtained for different models.

Introduction to Disease Prediction

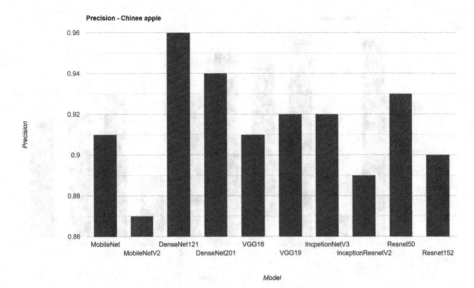

FIGURE 5.53 Precision of Chinee apple obtained for different models.

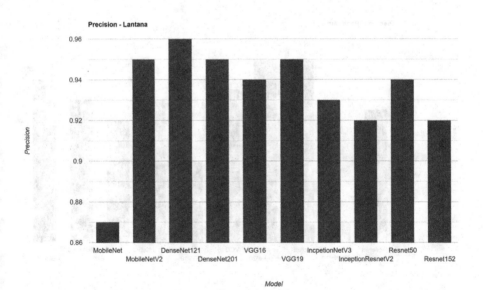

FIGURE 5.54 Precision of Lantana obtained for different models.

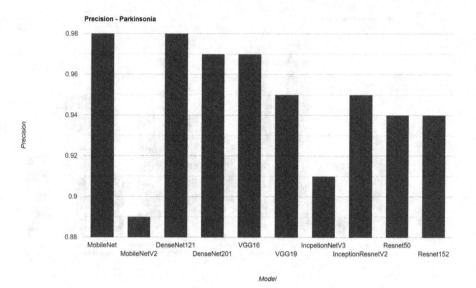

FIGURE 5.55 Precision of Parkinsonia obtained for different models.

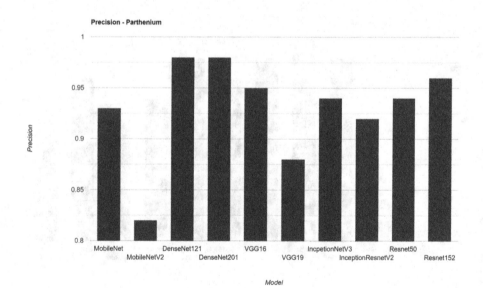

FIGURE 5.56 Precision of Parthenium obtained for different models.

Introduction to Disease Prediction

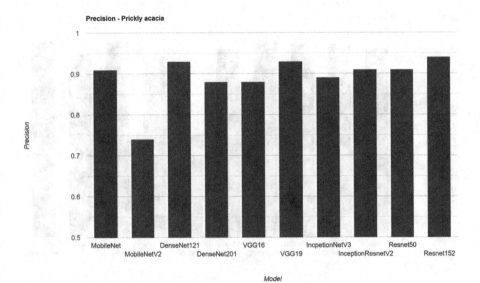

FIGURE 5.57 Precision of Prickly acacia obtained for different models.

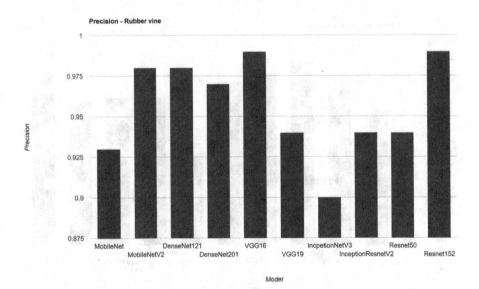

FIGURE 5.58 Precision of Rubber vine obtained for different models.

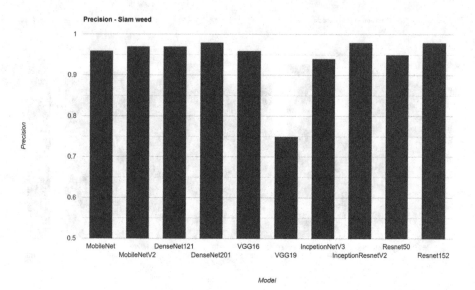

FIGURE 5.59 Precision of Siam weed obtained for different models.

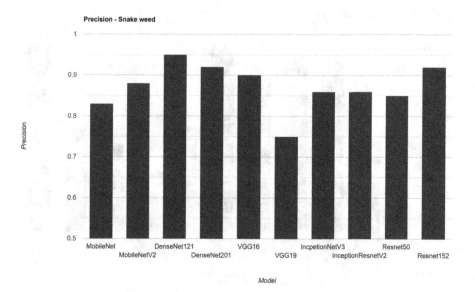

FIGURE 5.60 Precision of Snake weed obtained for different models.

FIGURE 5.61 Android application layout.

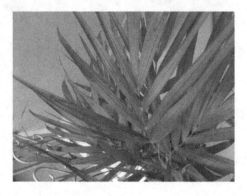

FIGURE 5.62 Result when a non-weed plant is uploaded.

Introduction to Disease Prediction

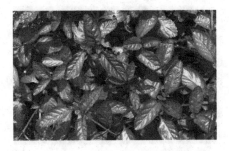

FIGURE 5.63 Result when Snake weed is uploaded.

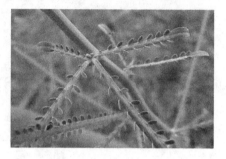

FIGURE 5.64 Result when Rubber vine is uploaded.

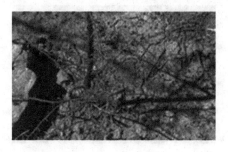

FIGURE 5.65 Result when Prickly acacia is uploaded.

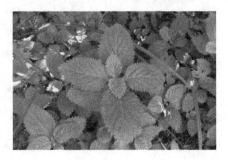

FIGURE 5.66 Result when Lantana is uploaded.

Introduction to Disease Prediction

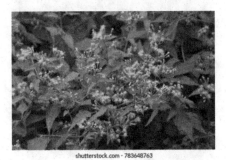

FIGURE 5.67 Result when Siam weed is uploaded.

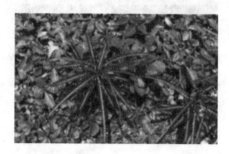

FIGURE 5.68 Result when Parkinsonia is uploaded.

Introduction to Disease Prediction

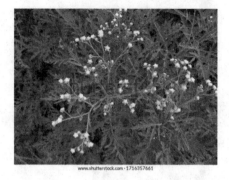

FIGURE 5.69 Result when Parthenium is uploaded.

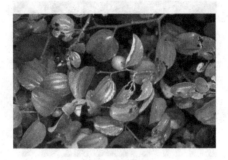

FIGURE 5.70 Result when Chinee apple is uploaded.

5.6 CONCLUSION AND FUTURE SCOPE

A comparison study of different deep learning based models for the detection and classification of weeds (9 classes) and crops has been done. One of the challenges faced was the lack of a good GPU configuration. This was overcome by using Google Colab Pro (a premium version of Google Colab with faster GPU and increased storage), which is a platform (cloud) specifically used for Python-based notebooks. Colab makes it very easy to use Keras and TensorFlow libraries.

After performing a comparative study of several deep learning based models implemented on an open-source dataset (DeepWeeds), it has been found that DenseNet121 gave the best accuracy (97%), F1 Score (0.97) and sensitivity (0.97).

To make this project accessible and understandable to everyone, a simple, easy to use mobile Android application that displays the weeds classification output after the user uploads an image of a plant has been implemented.

Integrating this project with hardware, that is, field robots, unmanned aerial vehicles or all-terrain vehicles, would facilitate weed management by spraying pesticides after real-time detection of weeds.

Another enhancement that could be made to this project is by obtaining datasets of more classes of weeds to ensure a wide range of weeds can be detected and identified thereby improving the efficacy of weed management.

REFERENCES

[1] L. Jacob, A. Patil, K. Patil, & K.S. Charumathi (2021). Weed detection in Indian fields and disease detection using convolutional neural network. *Semantic Scholar*, Corpus ID: 235803809.

[2] M. Dyrmann, A.K. Mortensen, H.S. Midtiby, & R.N. Jørgensen (2016). Pixel-wise classification of weeds and crops in images by using a fully convolutional neural network. *Semantic Scholar*, Corpus ID: 52084224

[3] Florian J. Knoll, Vitali Czymmek, Leif O. Harders, & Stephan Hussmann (2019). Real-time classification of weeds in organic carrot production using deep learning algorithms, *Computers and Electronics in Agriculture*, 167, ID: 105097, ISSN 0168-1699, https://doi.org/10.1016/j.compag.2019.105097

[4] S. Jeba Priya, G. Naveen Sundar, D. Narmadha, & Shamila Ebenezer (2019). Identification of weeds using HSV Color spaces and labelling with machine learning algorithms. *International Journal of Recent Technology and Engineering (IJRTE)*, 8(1), 1781–1786, May. ISSN: 2277-3878

[5] Radhika Kamath, Mamatha Balachandra, & Srikanth Prabhu (2020). Paddy crop and weed discrimination: A multiple classifier system approach. *International Journal of Agronomy*, 2020, 1–14. Article ID 6474536. https://doi.org/10.1155/2020/6474536

[6] Y. Chen, Z. Wu, B. Zhao, C. Fan, & S. Shi (2021). Weed and corn seedling detection in field based on multi feature fusion and support vector machine. *Sensors* 21, 212. https://doi.org/10.3390/s21010212

[7] R. Kingsy Grace, J. Anitha, R. Sivaramakrishnan, & M.S.S. Sivakumari (2021). Crop and Weed classification using deep learning. *Turkish Journal of Computer and Mathematics Education*, 12(7), 935–938.

[8] C.T. Selvi, R.S. Sankara Subramanian, & R. Ramachandran (2021). Weed Detection in Agricultural fields using Deep Learning Process, 7th International Conference on

Advanced Computing and Communication Systems (ICACCS), 2021, pp. 1470–1473, doi: 10.1109/ICACCS51430.2021.9441683

[9] Baydaulet Urmashev, Zholdas Buribayev, Zhazira Amirgaliyeva, Aisulyu Ataniyazova, Mukhtar Zhassuzak, and Amir Turegali (2021). Development of a weed detection system using machine learning and neural network algorithms (December 29, 2021). *Eastern-European Journal of Enterprise Technologies*, 6 (2(114)), 70–85. https://doi.org/10.15587/1729-4061.2021.246706, Available at SSRN: https://ssrn.com/abstract=4007300

[10] A. Subeesh, S. Bhole, K. Singh, N.S. Chandel, Y.A. Rajwade, K.V.R. Rao, S.P. Kumar, & D. Jat (2022). Deep convolutional neural network models for weed detection in polyhouse grown bell peppers. *Artificial Intelligence in Agriculture*, 6, 47–54. ISSN 2589-7217, https://doi.org/10.1016/j.aiia.2022.01.002

[11] Alaa Tharwat (2018). *Classification Assessment Methods: A Detailed Tutorial.* DOI: 10.1016/j.aci.2018.08.003

[12] Neha Verma, Sarita Kansal, Huned Malvi (2018). Development of native mobile application using android studio for cabs and some glimpses of cross platform apps. *International Journal of Applied Engineering Research* 13(16), 12527–12530. ISSN 0973-4562. © Research India Publications. www.ripublication.com

[13] A. Olsen, D.A. Konovalov, B. Philippa, et al. (2019). DeepWeeds: a multiclass weed species image dataset for deep learning. *Science Reports* 9, 2058. https://doi.org/10.1038/s41598-018-38343-3

[14] Masoud Mahdianpari, Bahram Salehi, Mohammad Rezaee, Fariba Mohammadimanesh, & Yun Zhang, (2018). Very deep convolutional neural networks for complex land cover mapping using multispectral remote sensing imagery. *Remote Sensing* 10, 1119. 10.3390/rs10071119

[15] Kaiming He, Xiangyu Zhang, Shaoqing Ren and Jian Sun (2015). Deep residual learning for image recognition. arXiv, abs/1512.03385

[16] K.S. Srujana, Sukruta N. Kashyap, G. Shrividhiya, C. Gururaj, & K.S. Induja (2022). Supply chain based demand analysis of different deep learning methodologies for effective covid-19 detection. 135–170, 10.1007/978-981-19-0240-6_9

[17] Zhixian Yang, Ruixia Dong, Hao Xu, & Jinan Gu (2020). Instance segmentation method based on improved mask R-CNN for the stacked electronic components. *Electronics* 9, 886. 10.3390/electronics9060886

[18] C. Szegedy, V. Vanhoucke, S. Ioffe, J. Shlens, & Z. Wojna (2016). Rethinking the Inception Architecture for Computer Vision. 2016 IEEE Conference on Computer Vision and Pattern Recognition (CVPR), pp. 2818–2826. doi: 10.1109/CVPR.2016.308

[19] Y. Bhatia, A. Bajpayee, D. Raghuvanshi, & H. Mittal, (2019). Image captioning using Google's inception-resnet-v2 and recurrent neural network. 2019 Twelfth International Conference on Contemporary Computing (IC3), pp. 1–6. doi: 10.1109/IC3.2019.8844921

[20] C.-Y. Lee, S. Xie, P. Gallagher, Z. Zhang, & Z. Tu. Deeplysupervised nets. In AISTATS, 2015.

[21] Karen Simonyan & Andrew Zisserman (2015). Very Deep Convolutional Networks for Large-Scale Image Recognition. https://doi.org/10.48550/arXiv.1409.1556

[22] M. Bansal, M. Kumar, M. Sachdeva, et al. (2021). Transfer learning for image classification using VGG19: Caltech-101 image data set. *Journal of Ambient Intelligent Human Computing*, 3609–3620. 10.1007/s12652-021-03488-z

[23] Brett Koonce (2021). ResNet 50. 10.1007/978-1-4842-6168-2 6

[24] Aswin Vellaichamy, Akshay Swaminathan, C. Varun, & S. Kalaivani (2021). Multiple plant leaf disease classification using densenet-121 architecture. *International Journal of Electrical Engineering and Technology.* 12, 38–57. 10.34218/IJEET.12.5.2021.005

[25] C. Gururaj (2018). Proficient Algorithm for features mining in fundus images through content based image retrieval. International Conference on Intelligent and Innovative Computing Applications (ICONIC), 108–113. 10.1109/ICONIC.2018.8601259

[26] V.N.A. Manaswi & Rizwan Patan (2022). A study on leaf image classification for plants using transfer learning. *Recent Patents on Engineering* 16. 10.2174/1872212116666220328123141

[27] C. Gururaj, D. Jayadevappa, & Satish Tunga. (2016). A study of different content based image retrieval techniques. 10.17148/IJARCCE.2016.5846

[28] Kanchan V Warkar (2021). A survey on multiclass image classification based on inception-v3 transfer learning model. *International Journal for Research in Applied Science and Engineering Technology* 9, 169–172. 10.22214/ijraset.2021.33018

[29] Prabhjot Kaur, Shilpi Harnal, Vinay Gautam, Mukund Singh, & Santar Pal Singh (2022). A novel transfer deep learning method for detection and classification of plant leaf disease. *Journal of Ambient Intelligence and Humanized Computing,* 1–18. 10.1007/s12652-022-04331-9

[30] K. Thaiyalnayaki Krishnan, & Christeena Joseph (2021). Classification of plant disease using SVM and deep learning. *Materials Today: Proceedings,* 47. 10.1016/j.matpr.2021.05.029

[31] Veena Nayak, Sushma P. Holla, K.M. Akshayakumar, & C. Gururaj. (2021). Machine learning methodology toward identification of mature citrus fruits. Computer Vision and Recognition Systems Using Machine and Deep Learning Approaches: Fundamentals, Technologies and Applications, 385–438. 10.1049/PBPC042E_ch16

[32] S. Sharanya, B.N. Raghuttama, B.R. Ananya, Simha R. Pranav, & C. Gururaj (2022). Deep Learning Based Plant Disease Detection. 10.1109/MysuruCon55714.2022.9972398

[33] Towhidul Islam, Nurul Absar, Abzetdin Z. Adamov, & Mayeen Uddin Khandaker (2021). *A Machine Learning Driven Android Based Mobile Application for Flower Identification.* Springer Nature Switzerland AG 2021. https://doi.org/10.1007/978-3-030-82269-9_13

[34] Convert TensorFlow models. www.tensorflow.org/lite/models/convert/convertmodels

[35] K.V.H. Avani, Deeksha Manjunath, & C. Gururaj. (2022) Deep Learning-Based Detection of Thyroid Nodules. *Multidisciplinary Applications of Deep Learning-Based Artificial Emotional Intelligence,* 107–135. IGI Global. DOI: 10.4018/978-1-6684-5673-6.ch008

6 Medical Record Management for Disease Management

Gururaj H. L., Soundarya Bidare Chandre Gowda and D. Basavesha

6.1 INTRODUCTION

The phrase 'medical records management' refers to a set of procedures and rules in charge of monitoring patient data throughout its entire lifetime. Even when it is created, a patient record needs to be properly kept, safeguarded, and maintained. The record must be properly destroyed after the required amount of time has passed. There is a complex system of regulations and standards governing the management of medical records, and for good reason. When medical records are handled incorrectly, patients are put in danger.

It has been demonstrated that hospitals' implementation of electronic health records increases patient safety, but poor management can lead to medication errors, missed diagnoses, treatment gaps, and other potentially lethal circumstances.

Another danger is with regard to patients' privacy. Highly sensitive personal information is present in medical records, and privacy is jeopardized when mistakes are made. Patients are losing faith due to an increase in healthcare data breaches. A recent consumer survey found that 87% of patients are reluctant to divulge their complete medical history due to worries about privacy regulations. Due to poor record-keeping, hospitals, medical practices, and other service providers could be subject to costly fines, legal action, and criminal accusations.

After a series of breaches exposed the health information of almost 79 million individuals, healthcare benefits provider Anthem agreed to pay the U.S. Department of Health and Human Services $16 million in 2016. Investigators from the government found that Anthem had violated the Health Insurance Portability and Accountability Act (HIPAA) by failing to take the necessary precautions to secure patient records.

Implementing electronic health records has the well-known effect of dividing medical records into two distinct skills. While administrative management deals with record governance outside of the treatment room, such as financing and insurance plans, the clinical medical record concentrates on condition management that is addressed in the treatment room. Further layers include socio-economic considerations, the patient's capacity for compliance with treatment, and decision-making abilities.

Many medical facilities now understand that their offices are more technologically equipped and have better communication tools than their patients. Chronic condition management (CCM), which is acknowledged as reimbursable by payers, as a new service as a result. CCM is a monthly service that users can use to maintain their medical records for a whole year. In essence, this service fulfills the newly added duty placed on patients to arrange their own medical data. People who have common to complex conditions that persist more than a year and could benefit from helping manage all the administrative tasks that go along with their disease are eligible for this service. CCM comprises everything that is medically related to the patient's health, including faxing, working together, doing business correspondence via email, documenting, and recording.

This was something that we thought was a great gift before the pandemic. However, this is a professional service that is carried out for the patient and recorded in the electronic health record of the particular medical practice. The drawback of this service is that ownership may change from year to year and storage may only be available to employees of that particular office. As a result, this service is constrained and shouldn't be used as a patient's primary source of emergency support.

6.2 CHARACTERISTICS OF CLINICAL RECORDS

A wide range of documents created by, or on behalf of, all the healthcare professionals involved in patient care are included in clinical records. This comprises: handwritten clinical notes, computerized/electronic clinical records, scanned records, and laboratory results.

There are several characteristics of clinical records:

1. Precisely prepares patients for the treatment of a given diagnosis
2. Reimbursable
3. Standard expectations for illness care and treatment direction
4. Advice based on data and strategies with a track record of success
5. Available in the treatment area
6. Definitive measured results

6.3 CHARACTERISTICS OF ADMINISTRATIVE RECORDS

Electronic data records known as administrative data are frequently created at the time of hospital discharge or the delivery of other services. They often include both primary and secondary diagnoses, as well as at least some details on treatments received and procedures carried out. They may include links to files that contain demographic data. Administrative statistics typically don't include clinical measurements like blood pressure or height and weight, or laboratory results like pathology or radiology reports.

The characteristics of administrative records are:

1. Helps the individual beyond the treatment room
2. Not reimbursable

3. When patients ask queries, nonstandard guidance is given
4. Advice drawn from personal experience
5. No definitive measure results

Learning how to construct a health record on your own can be difficult because many people, especially those who live in remote regions, lack access to the internet, fax machines, and a secure portal where professionals could comfortably communicate records. The core health advocacy competencies are shown in Table 6.1.

6.3.1 Types of Medical Records

Standard – A standard medical record is a compilation of notes and recordings made by a licensed practitioner to describe the history, diagnosis, course of treatment, or progress of one of their patients. Standard medical records are typically kept electronically and are only ever entered by a single practitioner at a specific point of service.

Non-standard – The entries, notes, recordings, and other standard records that are compiled by people who lack a medical licence, are not paid, and have not had professional training in healthcare constitute a non-standard (health) record. In a court of law, no one who contributed to this kind of record can be identified. Non-standard medical records, however, are significant and can be a very useful communication tool for the entire care team.

6.3.2 Tiers of Medical and Health Management

There are three tiers of medical and health management as shown in Figure 6.1.

TABLE 6.1
Core health advocacy competencies

Drivers	Patients Takeways
Increase treatment adherence	1. Possess less complications
	2. Fewer trips to the emergency department
	3. Higher quality appointments driven by information
	4. Minimize unanticipated expenses
Increase medical utilization	1. Enhanced readiness for medical appointments
	2. Decrease in pointless phone calls and office visits
Hone your risk management abilities	1. Make an accurate assessment of the services being delivered
	2. Better literacy and communication abilities in the health field
	3. Exposed to more advanced professional discourse
Efficiently handle medical records	1. Available health records as at the moment
	2. Preventing the loss of health data.
	3. On-demand documentation in physical copy for health information
	4. Information coordination between qualified offices

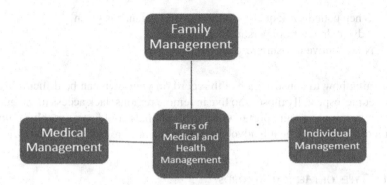

FIGURE 6.1 Tiers of health management.

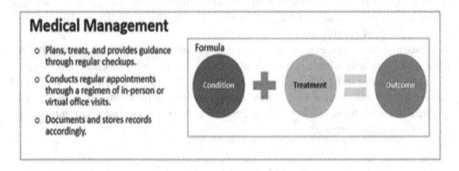

FIGURE 6.2 Medical management provider.

6.3.2.1 Medical Management

We may count on the provider to keep a record of the clinical data and services rendered as well as to give patients the necessary education in the treatment area. When medical management data are collected, they are often electronically kept inside. The majority of the leadership in charge of the medical management and treatment division belongs to your provider (Figure 6.2).

6.3.2.2 Individual Health Management

An initial audit of all health records is the final step in individual management. Create a cover page for yourself to start this process and work with pre-existing documents, or keep a record of

1. your special social circumstances (for example, your religion),
2. your way of life (for example, your job – if under special circumstances), and
3. your family and medical history (see Figure 6.3).

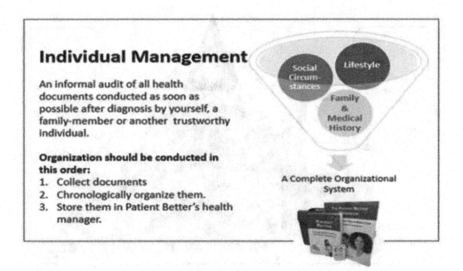

FIGURE 6.3 Individual medical management provider.

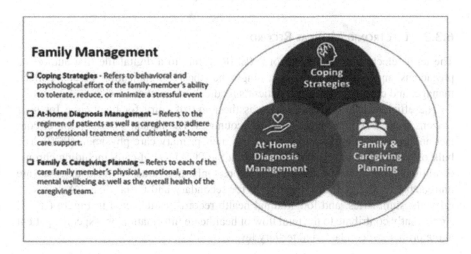

FIGURE 6.4 Family management.

6.3.2.3 Family Management

This is a three-pronged strategy for people with chronic, complex disorders to make sure that they and the family members who are caring for them are in the best physical, emotional, and mental health during the entire diagnosis process. It's important to be aware of who is assisting with planning, collaborating, and documenting one's care even though other people's health information shouldn't be included in the individual's health record (Figure 6.4).

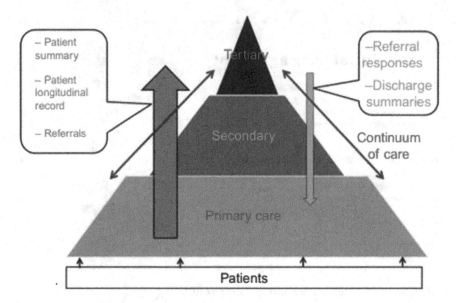

FIGURE 6.5 Healthcare information for health management.

6.3.3 Electronic Medical Record

The term 'electronic medical record' (EMR) refers to a digital file that authorised physicians and employees from a single healthcare organization create, collect, manage, and consult regarding a patient's medical information.

The efficient use of primary care as the point of entry for healthcare for their citizens is the essential success in many countries. The patient's initial point of contact and primary healthcare practitioner is their primary care physician (PCP). The bulk of healthcare concerns are managed at the PCP level of care, including chronic conditions like diabetes and hypertension. Only individuals whose diseases are untreatable by the PCP are referred on for secondary and tertiary care. As a result, referrals, summaries, and longitudinal health records, as depicted in Figure 6.5, all significantly contribute to the total flow of healthcare information on a specific patient at the primary, secondary, and tertiary levels.

6.3.4 Electronic Health Record

A compliant electronic medical record that adheres to recognized health information technologyinteroperability standards that is created, managed, and consulted by authorized medical professionals from diverse healthcare organizations. The idea of a person's longitudinal health record is represented by it. A single comprehensive longitudinal or lifetime record for a single patient is essentially created by combining many electronic medical records (EMRs) from various healthcare organizations. This requires the interoperability – the capacity of different EMRs to communicate data with one another – which is made possible by following a particular set of established

Medical Record Management for Disease Management

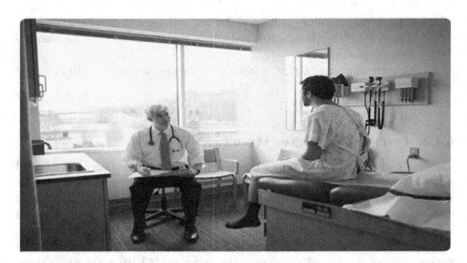

FIGURE 6.6 Educating patients.

coding methods. Examples include ICD-10 for diagnosis, LOINC for test data, and HL7 for communicating.

6.4 OVERVIEW OF DISEASE MANAGEMENT

A medical approach called disease management educates patients how to take care of their chronic illnesses. Patients are instructed to take ownership of knowing self-care. They gain knowledge on how to avoid prospective issues and the deterioration of their health.

Example – Teaching a diabetic patient about disease management involves showing them how to keep their blood sugar levels in check. The idea of teaching patients illness management was born out of a desire to enhance the calibre of a patient's care, as seen in Figure 6.6. In an effort to reduce healthcare expenses, health insurance firms moved their attention to illness management in 2005. If patients knew how to better care for their health conditions, the insurance company would save money.

6.4.1 COMPONENTS OF DISEASE MANAGEMENT

The below are the components identified by the Disease Management Association of America:

1. *Identify the target populations*: Determine which diseases should be addressed and how people suffering from those diseases can be enrolled in a disease management programme.
2. Create evidence-based best practices for the conditions that will be managed.
3. *Build collaborative practice models*: In addition to doctors, disease management programmes employ nurses, nutritionists, pharmacists, and other team members.

4. *Educate the patient*: In addition to doctors, additional team members such as nurses, dietitians, pharmacists, and others are also used in disease management programmes.
5. *Measure outcomes*: Create a system for tracking expenses, utilization, and health outcomes.
6. Reporting and feedback.

6.4.2 Effectiveness of Disease Management

The first studies on illness management-based cost control in late 2007 revealed that costs were not being managed. It was concerning that the main reason for implementing these programmes had not been accomplished. However, there were advantages to illness management programmes in terms of patient satisfaction and the enhancement of their quality of life.

People with diabetes or heart failure were the main target of the Medicare Health Support programme. According to a study that compared 163,107 patients with a control group, disease management programmes did not lower emergency department or hospital admissions. For these patients, there were no Medicare cost savings.

However, the Veterans Administration's randomized trial of disease management for chronic obstructive pulmonary disease discovered a decline in hospital admissions and emergency room (ER) visits as well as financial savings.

Systematic analyses of illness management initiatives have not consistently revealed cost reductions or better patient outcomes. This would indicate that disease management programmes need to be enhanced to achieve both objectives more successfully.

6.5 MEDICAL RECORDS DEPARTMENT: PLANNING, JOB AND FUNCTION

The organization and management of the medical records department (MRD) must be based on the principle that patients come first. The medical record department assists the patient by always ensuring that the records are accurate, accessible, and complete. In order to accomplish its intended goals, the work of the medical record department should be organized in accordance with its functions. Processing of outpatient and inpatient records, retrieval, record storage, and disease- and procedure-specific coding and indexing are among the duties of the department. In a smaller department with fewer personnel, it is preferable for all staff to be informed about every aspect of the medical record department in order to ensure that the department functions efficiently.

6.5.1 Planning the Work Environment

The planning function includes offering the medical records assistant a comfortable work environment. This entails planning ahead when selecting the location and size of a workplace, buying office supplies and equipment, and taking into account spatial conditioning factors like the right lighting and colour.

Medical Record Management for Disease Management

6.5.1.1 Location Prerequisites

The outpatient and inpatient care units' registration offices communicate regularly with the medical record department. Every day, a large number of doctors visit the medical records area to complete or examine their records. It is necessary to be close to the admission and discharge office, medical records department, and new and review registration counters.

If the medical records department is not staffed 24/7, it should be located close to the admitting or outpatient area so that hospital employees can easily access medical records in an emergency. Security monitoring for the preservation of equipment and patient data should also be considered when the department is closed.

6.5.1.2 Space Requirement

When allocating space, it is essential to take into account the departmental services to be provided, the tools and computer systems to be employed, and the daily workload to be managed. Despite the fact that hospital services vary somewhat from one another, the following services and tasks should be considered when allocating space: record filing cabins, coding and indexing desks, medical records sorting and arranging desks, outpatient registration areas, and admitting and discharge offices.

The space needed for the medical record service is frequently insufficient and causes a general issue. In order to avoid the excessively frequent filing issues in the medical records department, the space requirements should be regularly assessed by the medical records technician.

The medical records technician should set aside funds for future requirements and reserve the necessary space in advance of MRD's growth.

6.5.1.3 Equipment Requirement

Open-shelf file cabinets are the most typical type of storage solution for medical documents. They are more affordable. You can file or obtain records more rapidly with the aid of a medical records assistant. Most significantly, open shelves conserve space and let you store more books in a given amount of floor space. According to the figure, open-shelf filing equipment can have 7 or 10 shelves, with a height ranging from 9 to 12 feet. A single open-shelf filing unit can hold 5,250 records using seven open shelves that are each three feet long and one feet wide and have dividers to fit an average of 750 outpatient records in one compartment.

The best source of information for determining realistic estimations of the necessary quantity of space is a review of records from the last several years. It is feasible to determine the typical number of sheets per medical record for a patient who was released over the course of two or three months as well as for a follow-up clinic session. To do this, include the sheets used for the present episode of care and the sheets used for previous inpatient or outpatient sessions (Figure 6.7).

To expedite the retrieval, filing, and finding of documents, record dividers should be positioned throughout the files. The thickness of the bulk of the medical records in the shelves determines how many dividers are required. A divider for every 125 medical records is sufficient for medium-thick medical records. Durability and quality

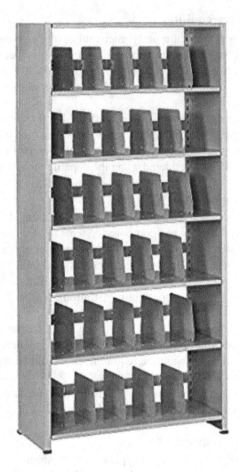

FIGURE 6.7 Open shelf filing unitRecord dividers between files.

should be your top priorities when buying dividers. The formula below may be used to calculate the total amount of dividers required:

$$\text{Total number of records} = \frac{\text{Total number of dividers}}{\text{Number of records between dividers}}$$

If the total number of records is unknown, a reasonable approximation can be made by multiplying the filing inches by the usual number of records per inch. A number of record shelves should be counted in order to get the average number of records per inch. To facilitate retrieval of the requested data in a healthcare facility, medical records should be stored and retained in the most effective way possible. Either centralization or decentralization may be used for the medical record file area.

Medical Record Management for Disease Management

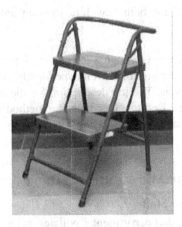

FIGURE 6.8 Step-type steel ladder.

6.5.1.4 Climbing Devices

In order to maximize the height of the filing cabinet for medical records, an open shelf filing unit was created. It could be challenging to extract medical records that are stacked higher than 5 or 6 feet. As a result, hospitals use a variety of climbing tools to access the medical data that are kept up to 8 or 9 feet in the air (Figure 6.8).

To conveniently file or recover the documents, a step ladder or an aluminium ladder with a rubber bush at the bottom of the leg will be more useful to the retriever. A lightweight aluminium ladder will be simple to transport inside the medical records area. The rubber bush prevents the ladder from falling.

As seen in Figure 6.8, the step-type steel ladder will be simple for women to ascend. Climbing equipment will therefore be significantly more beneficial for the file assistants to quickly deposit or retrieve medical data while preventing unneeded mishaps.

6.5.1.5 Organizational Chart

Each employee needs to be aware of the boundaries of his or her power and duty, and an organizational chart is a useful tool for explaining these relationships to others. It is important to design a clear organizational chart with the roles and lines of authority shown. This will guarantee that neither the chain of command nor the roles of the staff members are unclear. For any task carried out in a medical records department, procedures might be written.

6.5.1.6 Job Description

Written procedure manual for job description provides a valuable tool for two reasons.

1. It provides a clear understanding of what is expected of a worker who frequently executes a procedure.

2. It is a useful tool for both new hire training and cross-training existing personnel.

An employee should be guided through a technique by a medical record technician at least once before attempting to follow it independently. Additionally, all staff must have precise job descriptions. The job description for the employees who carry out the operation should be revised together with the method itself. The qualifications necessary for an individual to execute a job satisfactorily are detailed in their job description.

6.5.2 Functions of the Medical Records Department

6.5.2.1 Training of New Staff

Written notice of hospital and departmental policies, rules, and procedures must be provided to every new hire. A staff member cannot be held responsible for their acts unless they are aware of what is expected of them by their supervisor.

6.5.2.2 Provide On-Job Orientation and Training

All employees have the right to thorough training for the job to which they are assigned. All new departmental staff should receive three to four weeks of intensive training before being placed on their own.

The new employee should initially be introduced to the entire department's staff before moving on to the key hospital departments that work closely with the medical record department. Employees members should be put under an experienced medical records supervisor during the initial training phase. This supervisor will then provide 'on the job training' and advise the new staff in adhering to the proper policies and procedures.

6.5.2.3 Evaluate Performance

Performance reviews ought to be conducted on a regular basis. Make the employees aware of your talents and weaknesses.

The medical records technician ought to help the employees improve subpar work. The supervisor and the medical records technician should collaborate on the goal-setting process. This gives a staff member direction for professional growth, fosters job satisfaction, and boosts self-assurance. It is unacceptable to verbally reprimand a staff member in front of other people.

Staff members should be encouraged to offer comments, and supervisors should work to maintain two-way communication with them. Supervisors themselves ought to be understanding while hearing about staff members' issues. In order to get a job done by the team or to solve a problem, a manager occasionally needs to provide priority.

Medical Record Management for Disease Management

6.5.2.4 Main Functions
The main functions of medical records department are

1. Out-patient service
   - enrollment of new and returning patients
   - directing a patient to various facilities and specialties
   - medical records for both inpatients and outpatients are coded.
   - gathering, handling, classifying, and organizing medical records
2. In-patient service
   - Admitting patients
   - Discharging patients

6.5.2.5 Out-patient
The registration of new and returning patients and their referral for evaluation and treatment to the appropriate departments or specializations are the duties of the out-patient service area.

6.5.2.6 New and Revisit Registration
The new registration area's medical records assistant carries out the following duties:

I. Procedure for new registration
   - Before enrolling new patients, the medical records assistant first checks the new registration counter for the sociological data form, outpatient records, and a plastic pouch to hold ID cards, staplers, and bell pins.
   - The medical records assistant makes sure the system and other instruments are in good working order by checking them.
   - The counter for new registration opens in the morning.
   - The patient's name, age, sex, and name of any close relatives are all listed on the sociological form, along with the patient's address and city, phone number(s), mobile phone number(s), and fax number.
   - At the new registration counter, the completed sociological data form is gathered and reviewed for any errors, omissions, or amendments.
   - The data is subsequently input into the system by the medical records assistant.
   - The patient is asked to pay any fees associated with the new registration.
   - The false note identifying machine is then used to ensure that the currency notes are genuine.
   - The medical record assistant asks the patient if there have been any letters of recommendation from other doctors.
   - The patient receives an identification card displaying his medical record number along with a receipt.
   - The patient is aware of how long his appointment with the doctor is expected to go. The patient and his outpatient record are then taken to the doctor for a consultation.

II. Procedure for revisit registration
- Patients who return to the hospital after their fresh registration the next day are referred to as revisit patients.
- The medical records assistant makes sure everything at the counter is operating properly by testing the system and other equipment.
- The counter for revisit registration opens in the morning.
- The patient who is returning presents their identity card at the registration desk.
- The medical records assistant then registers the patient in the system by entering the patient's medical record number.
- The date of registration and the medical records number are entered on the tracer card to prepare it for record retrieval. When medical records are not located where they should be, the tracer card's job is to assist the retriever in finding them.
- The tracer card is retained after retrieving the medical record using the MR Number.

2. Procedure for patient guides
- As part of their training in maintaining medical records, trainees are given the responsibility of serving as patient guides.
- The patient guide's job is to direct patients from the new and updated registration area to the relevant units.
- After registration, the public address system calls the new and returning patients who are waiting in the lounge.
- The patient guides will direct them to the appropriate units and specialties after verifying the patient's names and the city.

6.5.2.7 Processing of Out-patient and In-patient Medical Records

The main functions of this area are:

- Gathering of medical records from the discharge counter, specialty clinics, and outpatient clinics
- Examining patient and outpatient records for errors
- Coding in the system of completed records
- Sorting and placing medical records in a sequential order

6.5.2.8 Collection and Sorting Out of Disposed of Records for Filing

- The patient guides retrieve the patient medical documents from each outpatient clinic's trash box, specialty clinic's disposal box, and discharge counter.
- Outpatient and inpatient records are examined for deficiencies in the obtained medical records. The final diagnosis, the doctor's signature, and any incompleteness are checked in the medical records.
- The medical records are then divided into groups and put in the ascending order before being filed in various medical record boxes.
- Each medical record box has a serial number issued to it in a continuous series ranging from 1 to 10,000, 10001 to 20,000, and so on.

- A medical records assistant is assigned to file each medical record box on the appropriate rack.

6.5.2.9 In-patient Service
Two elements make up the in-patient medical record services. Both the Accident and Emergency (casualty) Service and the Admission and Discharge Counter are involved.

6.5.2.10 Admission Counter
The entire year, this admissions desk is open 24 hours a day. For the following tasks, staff are assigned in two shifts (morning and night).

- After counselling for their preferred room and lens type, patients are led by the counsellors to the admission counter.
- The employee at the admissions desk takes payment for the procedure, and the system generates an advance receipt.
- The staff signs the receipt before giving it to the patient.
- On the operation consent form, the patient's or his attendant's signature is required.
- All of the patient's pertinent medical record forms are kept in a coloured folder. The specialty to which the patient has been admitted is indicated by this folder.
- The nursing team then transports the patient and the surgical case sheet to the ward or theatre.

6.5.2.11 In-patient Coding Assistant
- The inpatient coding assistant receives the medical records following the operation in the operating room.
- Each medical record is coded for the surgery carried out in the operating room, which causes the system's charges for the operation to be updated automatically.
- During the course of the surgery, if the patient needs a monitor or if any other additional procedures are performed, they are likewise charged and updated in the system.

6.5.2.12 Discharge Counter
- The nursing staff delivers the case document to the discharge counter after receiving it from the ward.
- The final receipt is generated according to the number of days stay and for the surgery performed
- The staff at the discharge counter informs the patient of the follow-up date for their subsequent visit.

6.5.2.13 Departmental Meetings
Weekly general meetings with all departmental workers should be held to examine the daily operations of the medical records department. The staff members can be informed of any fresh ideas developed for the department's betterment. The medical records technician can discuss staff and departmental difficulties and concerns with

the employees, and a suitable solution should be found to ensure the department's efficient operation.

There must be more than just skilled technicians working in the medical records department. In order to create a discipline that is effective and well-organized, he or she must be both a leader and an innovator. To stay current with developments in both medicine and data recording and retrieval technology, constant effort is required. The administration and organization of the medical record department effectively play a key role in the certification of healthcare institutions. The medical records department of the healthcare facility is in charge of maintaining the accuracy, confidentiality, and accessibility of the patient's medical record at all times. Only when it is appropriately controlled and organized by the medical records assistant can it carry out these duties.

6.5.2.14 Key Points to Remember
- It is important to keep in mind that the proper care of the sick and injured is the primary obligation and goal of any health facility.
- With the exception of the specifically trained and supervisory employees, a monthly job roster must be created and the staff should be rotated from one division or unit to another.
- Every employee's job description should be documented explicitly, and an organizational chart outlining the roles and lines of power should be constructed.
- It is recommended to hold regular weekly meetings with all departmental workers to go over the daily tasks completed by the medical records department.
- Staff members should be assigned to a medical records supervisor with expertise during the initial training phase. This supervisor must then provide 'on the job training' and assist the new hire in adhering to the proper policies and procedures.
- For effective management, cooperative and responsible employees are crucial.

6.6 HEALTHCARE DATA BREACHES

Healthcare is very delicate and private. One of the most offensive sorts of data breaches is when a person's medical history or current treatments are made public due to a breach in healthcare data. Hackers get access to information through healthcare breaches that they can use to steal identities and carry out their data theft missions. There are numerous common elements that raise the danger of healthcare breaches, just like there are with other cybersecurity attacks. These consist of:

- *Outdated systems*: The most sophisticated data is kept by healthcare companies, and frequently, this data is maintained in incredibly out-of-date systems. Some systems are never modified or are altered after a breach because it can be expensive to update or switch to systems with better protection. They are susceptible to attacks because their security procedures are outdated and inefficient.
- *Poor testing*: An inactive security strategy is less effective than one that regularly conducts testing for vulnerabilities and penetration.
- *Assuming there is no risk*: The notion that HIPPA regulations provide sufficient security does not protect healthcare organizations or the individuals they serve.

For instance, HIPPA does not mandate encryption despite the fact that it might be a useful tool for safeguarding consumer data.

6.6.1 Protecting Patients Data from Data Breaches

Healthcare data breaches are costly for the companies they affect as well as for the patients who must seek to recover their data.

Measures healthcare providers are implementing to protect patients include:

- Plans for incident response to help businesses swiftly locate, stop, and lessen the effects of breaches.
- Utilization of backup generators for healthcare system compromise and power outages, as well as the usage of cloud-based systems, which are still relatively new in the field of healthcare but offer crucial backup of patient records in the event of a breach.
- Data encryption techniques for data at rest and data in motion are compliant with National Institute of Standards and Technology standards.
- Training for staff on how to access, use, and protect patient data.
- Protection against data loss, including sharing files with authorization and evaluating the security architecture

Between 2009 and 2021, the HHS Office for Civil Rights received 4,419 instances of medical data breaches involving 500 or more records. A total of 314,063,186 healthcare records have been lost, stolen, disclosed, or illegitimately shared as a result of these breaches. That will represent more than 94.63% of the U.S. population in 2021. Figure 6.9 shows that in 2018, reports of healthcare data breaches affecting 500 or more records were made on average once every day. After only four years, the

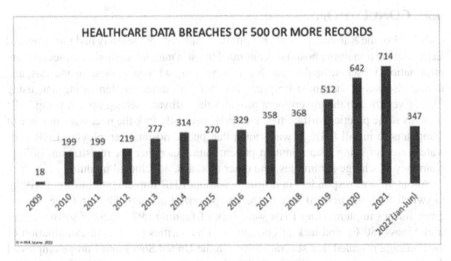

FIGURE 6.9 Healthcare data breaches between 2009 and 2021.

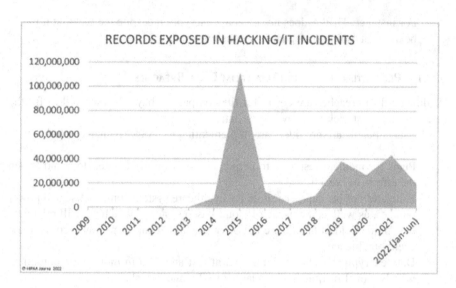

FIGURE 6.10 Records exposed in hacking between 2009 and 2022.

rate had doubled. Healthcare data breaches involving 500 or more records per day on average were reported 195 times in 2021.

Figure 6.10 depicts the total number of records exposed in hacking incidents between 2009 and 2022. A large number of records were exposed between 2014 and 2016.

Table 6.2 depicts the healthcare information which is breached in the year 2016. This table also gives the information about what is the cause for the healthcare data breach and total number of records exposed.

6.7 CONCLUSION

Only 23% of the Karnataka public hospitals considered for the study had implemented EHR, and the remaining hospitals continued to use a manual method to protect patient information. Observational research was done along with questionnaire analysis, and it was discovered that most hospitals had not yet started implementing and using EHR. Even though the government provides the software, setting up and using EHR presents some practical difficulties. Hospitals generally lack the necessary number of computers to install EHR. It was shown that public hospitals employing EHR software were not using it to maintain patient data, but rather for registration, billing, pharmacy, discharge summaries, and other modules, not clinical modules.

About 96% of responders in hospitals without EHR implementation were willing to switch from the manual way to the computerized method. The top three reasons given for not implementing EHR were lack of funding (5%), lack of software user friendliness (80%), and lack of consent from authorities (15%). An examination of the literature revealed that several nations in the United States and Europe employed the strategy of providing additional incentives to doctors who used EHRs during the

TABLE 6.2
Healthcare data breaches of 2016

Rank	Covered Entity	Entity Type	Cause of Breach	Records Expos
1	Banner Health	Healthcare Provider	Hacking/IT incident	3,620,000
2	Newkirk Products Inc.	Business Associate	Hacking/IT incident	3,466,120
3	21st Century	Healthcare Provider	Hacking/IT incident	2,213,597
4	Valley Anesthesiology Consultants	Healthcare Provider	Hacking/IT incident	882,590
5	Count of Los Angeles Departments of Health and Mental Health	Healthcare Provider	Hacking/IT incident	749,017
6	Bon Secours Health System Incorporated	Healthcare Provider	Unauthorized access/Disclosure	651,971
7	Peachtree Orthopedic Clinic	Healthcare Provider	Hacking/IT incident	531,000
8	Radiology Regional center PA	Healthcare Provider	Loss	483,063
9	Califomia Correctional health care services	Healthcare Provider	Theft	400,000
10	Community Health plan of Washington	Healthcare Plan	Hacking/IT incident	381,504

early phases of EHR introduction. This approach was only employed up until the advent of EHRs. It has been shown that it is highly challenging to give incentives for the use of EHRs in India, hence it would be beneficial to make EHR usage mandatory in hospitals.

Our findings from this study lead us to advise hospitals to adopt user-friendly and secure EHR software. Provide users with enough training so they feel confident using it consistently and electronically recording all health observations. For efficient use of EHRs, a good IT infrastructure and support system are absolutely necessary.

BIBLIOGRAPHY

Andieh, S.O., Yoon-Flannery, K., Kuperman, G.J., Langsam, D.J., Hyman, D., Kaushal, R. Challenges to EHR implementation in electronic- versus paper-based office practices. *Journal of General Internal Medicine* 23(6) (2008): 755–761. https://doi.org/10.1007/s11606-008-0573-5

Anupama, R., Pahwa, M. Hospital information management systems (HIMS) – A study of efficacy in Indian scenario. *Amity Management Review*, 3(1) (2013): 40–49.

Collins, F.S., Varmus, H. A new initiative on precision medicine. *New England Journal of Medicine* 372(9) (2015): 793–795.

Dai, L., Gao, X., Guo, Y., Xiao, J., Zhang, Z. Bioinformatics clouds for big data manipulation, *Biol. DirectBiol Direct*, 7(1) (2012): 43.

Epstein, R.S., Sherwood, L.M. From outcomes research to disease management: a guide for the perplexed. *Annals of Internal Medicine*. 124(9) (1996): 832–837.

Fernandez, A.R., Crowe, R.P., Bourn, S. et al. COVID-19 preliminary case series: characteristics of EMS encounters with linked hospital diagnoses. *Prehospital Emergency Care* 25(1) (2020): 16–27. Epub 2020 Jul 31.

Geissbuhler, A., Safran, C., Buchan, I., et al. Trustworthy reuse of health data: a transnational perspective. *International Journal of Medical Informatics* 82 (2013) :1–9.

Ginter, P.M., Duncan, J., Swayne, L.E. (2018). *The Strategic Management of Healthcare Organizations*. John Wiley & Sons.

Grant, R.W., Middleton, B. Improving primary care for patients with complex chronic diseases: can health information technology play a role? *CMAJ* 181(1–2) (2009): 17–18.

Huang, L., Lan, X., Fang, P., An, J., Min, Wang, F. Promises and challenges of big data computing in health sciences, *Big Data Research*, 2(1) (2015): 2–11.

Hussein, Ahmed F., et al. A medical records managing and securing blockchain based system supported by a genetic algorithm and discrete wavelet transform. *Cognitive Systems Research* 52 (2018): 1–11.

Kasthuri, A. Challenges to healthcare in India – The five A's. *Indian Journal of Community Medicine* 43(3) (2018): 141–143. doi: 10.4103/ijcm.IJCM_194_18. PMID: 30294075; PMCID: PMC6166510.

McMullen, C.K., Schneider, J., Altschuler, A., Grant, M., Hornbrook, M.C., Liljestrand, P., Krouse, R.S. Caregivers as healthcare managers: health management activities, needs, and caregiving relationships for colorectal cancer survivors with ostomies. *Supportive Care in Cancer* 22(9) (2014): 2401–2408.

Medical Record Management 101 | Oversee Care Like an Expert (patientbetter.com)

Mishra, A., Jaiswal, A., Chaudhari, L., Bodade, V. Health record management system – A web-based application. *Journal of ISMAC*. 3 (2022): 301–313. 10.36548/jismac.2021.4.002.

Mosadeghrad, A.M. Factors influencing healthcare service quality. *International Journal of Health Policy Management* 3(2) (2014): 77–89. doi: 10.15171/ijhpm.2014.65. PMID: 25114946; PMCID: PMC4122083.

Nehemiah, L. Towards EHR interoperability in Tanzania hospitals: Issues, challenges and opportunities. *International Journal of Computer Science, Engineering and Applications*, 4(4) (2014): 29–36. https://doi.org/10.5121/ijcsea.2014.4404

Prados-Suarez, B., Molina, C., Peña-Yañez, C. Providing an integrated access to EHR using electronic health records aggregators. *Student Health Technology Informatics* 270 (2020): 402–406.

Wong, R.E.X., Bradley, Elizabeth H. Developing patient registration and medical records management system in Ethiopia. *International Journal for Quality in Health Care* 21.4 (2009): 253–258.

Yan, Y., Qin, X., Wu, Y., Zhang, N., Fan, J., Wang, L. A restricted Boltzmann machine based two-lead electrocardiography classification. In Proc. 12th Int. Conf. Wearable Implantable Body Sens. Netw., June 2015, pp. 1–9.

7 Prediction Models for Health Care

Kiran, M. S. Hemanth Kumar, D. S. Sunil Kumar, M. T. Ganesh Kumar and S. Nandini

7.1 INTRODUCTION

Different behavior of brain cells can cause different abnormalities, which include anaplasia, atypia, neoplasia and necrosis, leading to brain tumor [1]. Brain tumor may or may not be symptomatic so they can be detected by symptoms exhibited by patients or can be identified on computed tomographic (CT) scan or magnetic resonance image (MRI) impressions [2]. According to the World Health Organization, brain tumor was detected in more than 22,000 patients in the United States in 2016. "National Brain Tumor Society estimates that every year 13000 patients die and 29000 patients suffer from primary brain tumors" [2, 3]. The World Health Organization reports states that there are 120 types of brain tumors that can be differentiated on the basis of size, shape, location, and characteristics of brain tissue [4–6]. Gliomas and glioblastomas are the most common type of brain tumors among others [7, 8]. Gliomas are further differentiated into two as low-grade gliomas (LGG) and as high-grade gliomas (HGG) [6, 9] whereas glioblastomas are more severe, life threatening and more frequent in adults aged between 40 and 50 years [3]. The average life expectancy of HGG patient is 14 months. Brain tumors are scaled from grade I to IV and they are further classified as benign (classes I and II) and malignant (classes III and IV) [2]. Benign tumors are non-aggressive and mostly they don't move from their infected area, whereas malignant tumors are aggressive and more fatal than benign tumors. They can grow enormously large and can move to any part of the body. Benign tumors are treatable through chemotherapy and they can be reduced to a smaller size [7]. They can be reduced to an extent where it can be removed through an operation. On the other hand, malignant tumors are non-operable, but they can be reduced through chemotherapy to some extent [7]. It may increase the life expectancy of the patient up to two or three months, but it is not completely curable [6, 7]. MR images are used to identify the type of brain tumor. Benign tumors are basically confined to one specific area and they do not explicitly harm the structure of the brain [3]. The MR image is converted into greyscale image where the white part of the image describes the infected portion and greyscale

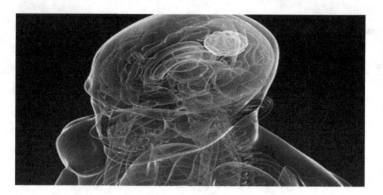

FIGURE 7.1 Brain tumor location in the brain.

portion shows the normal part of the brain. Detection of a benign tumor is relatively difficult compared to the detection of a malignant tumor [1, 4]. The reason behind it is that abnormality of the structure of the brain cannot be declared as benign tumor. The structure of a normal brain can be different from the average structure without any reason. Identification and detecting the exact size, location and age of a brain tumor is solely dependent on the skills and expertise of the radiologist. Manual detection and classification of the brain tumor includes a lengthy manual procedure adopted by the radiologist with chances of human errors. Image processing can be applied with the help of machine learning algorithms [5]. Automated detection and segmentation of a brain tumor is less time consuming, precise and yields efficient results [10]. Generative models [4] rely heavily on prior knowledge and use more of hand engineered components like support vector machine (SVM) and other feature extraction techniques [2, 5, 8]. Discriminative models have little prior knowledge and learn from the data given like neural networking, specifically convolutional neural network (CNN), which is an efficient approach [2, 4, 11]. CNN is a cutting-edge method used for object and edge detection in images. In this chapter, after minimal preprocessing on MR images, CNN is applied as an approach to train an effective system which can identify and classify a brain tumor [2, 4, 6]. CNN is a layered structure which involves kernels or filters that work in a pipeline method to extract multiple complex features [6, 10]. SoftMax is then applied to further obtain detailed results. In order to build an efficient and healthy system, training data was augmented and properly labelled [3, 6, 7]. Figure 7.1 shows the brain tumor location in the brain.

7.2 RELATED WORKS

Automation of brain tumor detection via machine learning has grown exponentially over the past decade [4]. The information we get from reading the related research papers that this proposed method has reached the implementation phase in some regions. As there is always room for improvement, some of the advanced algorithms for the solution of this problem are still under process. Most of the researchers have focused their work and proposed their techniques by using specific two kinds of models: generative models and discriminative models. These models are yet to be improvised, but they are giving promising results. On the elaboration of generative models, preprocessing, feature extraction and classification are the main steps. The most challenging task is the tissue appearance of the brain. Generative models are used to detect a brain tumor because of the abnormality of the tissue structure. The problem is that the tissue structure of a normal brain can differ from an average brain structure. This does not mean that a person has a tumor. It could be a simple deviation [7]. For finding the abnormality, biased field correction is proposed [12, 13].

Techniques like SoftMax and converting magnetic resonance images into greyscale are used by some researchers, but it is not a highly recommended method [1]. To overcome these challenging tasks, powerful techniques like SVM, discrete wavelet form (DWT) and Berkeley wavelet transformation (BWT) are used for the detection process [2, 13, 14]. For the segmentation of brain MRI, fuzzy c-means algorithm is used [2]. FCM can be further improvised for segmenting the data into homogeneous regions by using canny edge detection and BCET [15]. Preprocessing by the methods of skull stripping algorithms approach yields faster segmentation speed time due to K-means clustering and more accuracy because of fuzzy C-means algorithm [16, 17]. After segmentation, BWT is used for the extraction of the desired features. Furthermore, it is also used for reducing the feature complexity in order to make it easy for the understanding of the system [2]. Fuzzy C-means algorithm is also used for denoising the MRI by some of the researchers [6]. K-mean clustering and kernel expansion algorithms are used in generative models for the reclassification and removing the false positives [12]. SVM algorithm is then applied on the desired segmented results for the detection of a brain tumor [2]. The idea of the comparison of multiple segmented data and comparing their results was also proposed for achieving high levels of accuracy [18]. Moreover, SVM is also used for pre-processing of the MRI and normalizing the intensities using bias field correction. Image normalization using N4ITK method, feature extraction and data augmentation are also implied for the differentiation between LGG and HGG. After this process, extremely randomized forest is applied for the efficient training and testing of dataset [8]. For further improvements, cross-validation is used for better classification of the dataset [19]. Figure 7.2 shows the brain cancer cells present in the brain tumor image.

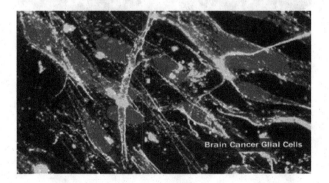

FIGURE 7.2 Brain tumor glial cells.

In addition to algorithms, canny edge detection, watershed transform, sobel operation, threshold algorithm, closed control algorithm, and object separation are also used. Having less false edges and closed contours, contour algorithms provide better results than sobel algorithms [21]. Based on abnormality maps and local texture, researchers have also proposed a new algorithm for automated brain tumor segmentation. Limited dataset with T1 and FLAIR is contrast enhanced, which is used for abnormality maps and local texture. For high-grade glioma detection, Random forest classification and voxel clustering are used [22]. Visual inspection of the results often shows over segmentation, which decreases the score. For discriminative models, we have studied different papers on neural network structures. DNN classifier provides high accuracy with convenient time rather than other traditional classifiers [1, 5]. For the segmentation through CNN architecture, a two-phase training of the dataset is carried out, which detects the tumor within a short range of time (i.e. 25 s to 3 min max) [4]. The effect of neurons on the brain tumor is shown in Figure 7.3.

Data augmentation was done on the datasets for increasing the number of inputs. So, more precise and accurate results can be achieved. NYUL method was applied for pixel intensity distribution. 3*3 kernel CNN is proposed for less weight and computational load. In the training set, data is augmented to detect rarer LGG by augmenting more HGG [22]. Random Forest algorithm has been very helpful and efficient in the 3D CNN image segmentation and a small kernel filter makes its results accurate and less expensive. It uses CNN to segment brain tumor into three layers with small size filter and Random Forest is applied to convert the data into 50 small subtress trees to analyze for the deep detection of the tumor [7, 11]. Moreover, other algorithms like KNN and CRF are also very productive. 2CNET, 3CNET and EnsambleNet of deep CNN are used for generating CNN and Incremental XCNet as an algorithm is used. The proposed CNN for hyper parameters is a unique approach as algorithm ELOBA-lambda is used for the iteration. The proposed three methods are high end and with their combination yield a high result of 0.88, 0.87, 0.89 within 20.87 s approximately [3]. Another algorithm that is being used is Hough-CNN. Different CNN architectures are evaluated, with varying number of kernels, CNN parameters and layers using limited data and limited computational resources. Hough-CNN outperformed Voxel-wise

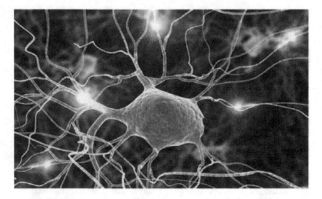

FIGURE 7.3 Brain tumor neuron effects.

segmentation of other CNN structures, while using limited dataset and limited computational resources. Furthermore Hough-CNN does not need post-processing [10]. 2D and 3D CNN are used separately for the classification and segmentation of brain tumor through automation, which is more efficient than supervised learning. First, patch is generated through MR image and CNN is performed on that generated patch. A model is being trained by the process of striding, padding, max pooling, connected layer, ReLU and SoftMax. DNN-based architecture is applied on the dataset of 384, which, produces promising results on the BRATS Benchmark [23]. Researchers have used CNN approach with a two-fold validation. Results for each fold are evaluated by a CNN architecture, which was trained on another fold. To some context, they used previous methods like randomized forests (RF) to double the amount of training data as compared to CNN. Evaluated results indicate that the CNN architecture is already capable of achieving high accuracy results [24]. Usually pipeline approach is used for pre-processing but automatic detection and segmentation is handled by deep learning methods in which different CNN approaches are used. This paper further gives a tabular comparison of different CNN approaches and their detection rate [20]. Bias field correction (N4TIK) method is used for intensity normalization. Flat blobs regions are removed by CCL algorithm. The augmentation of the images is done in this step by rotation, edge detection, flipping and such parameters to increase the size of dataset. VGG-19 architecture is used for the classification of the dataset; this architecture consists of 19 weighted layers [25]. For segmentation on multi-level information, Deep Medic is extended into multi-level deep medic [26]. Deep learning approach can also be applied in a way that trains the model using 2D patches and slices. It integrates FCNN and CRF and obtains three respective views. Then those results are combined by a vote fusion strategy [27]. Genetic algorithm can also

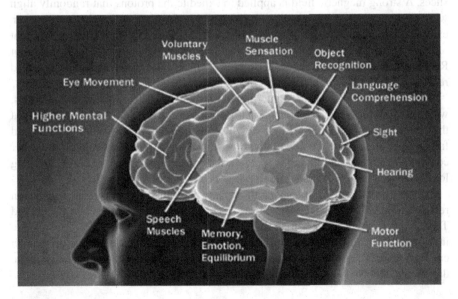

FIGURE 7.4 Brain function.

be used for improvising CNN architecture to produce better results. Deep learning features are not required for the feature extraction [9]. The authors of the works listed [28–31] increased the residual connection to dense connection in accordance with DenseNet. Even while a dense connection design appears to be more suitable for gradient back-propagation, the intricate close connection topology may need several memory operations while the network is being trained. Deep learning features are required for the feature extraction and tumor detection explained [32–34].

7.3 PROPOSED METHODOLOGY

We didn't come up with a brand-new solution to this issue. We think we have a little different strategy that is superior. Both generative and discriminative models will be used. For the purpose of tumor detection, generative models will be utilized and discriminative models would be applied for MRI segmentation. Figure 7.5 depicts a flow diagram for the segmentation and classification of brain tumors.

7.3.1 Preprocessing

The visualization, interpretation and evaluation of brain tumor is done by using non-invasive technique called MRI, which facilitates anatomical details of human brain in all planes such as axial, sagittal and coronal. MRI is efficient as compared to CT scan due to various reasons. First, it provides directions of blood flow in the human brain as well as vascular information. Second, it generates a series of brain slices without interference of extreme ionized radiations. Different functions of the brain are shown in Figure 7.4.

MRI uses magnetized characteristics of atomic nuclei to produce a series of brain slices. A strong magnetic field is applied to expedite the protons that randomly align with water content or atomic nuclei present in brain tissues. For this purpose, an external radio frequency (RF) is used, which excite the nuclei to pass through different relaxation times. A series of brain slices are created by changing the progression of RF pulses. The amount of time between the consecutive pulse sequence is called repetition time (TR). Table 7.1 gives the statistical features of different MRI images.

The human brain tissues are interpreted on the basis of two different categories, which rely on transverse and relaxation time and can easily be identified by looking at the cerebrospinal fluid (CSF). In T1-weighted images, the water content is darker and fatty tissues are brighter. While on the other hand, in T2-weighted images, the water content is brighter as compared to fat tissues and these images are generated by using long repetition time (TR) and time to echo (TE).

Along with T1 and T2 images, a third sequence called fluid attenuated inversion recovery (FLAIR) sequence is also used. It looks like T2 images, except its TR and TE relaxation times are very long as compared to T2. The sequence is very valuable in radiology because it helps to distinguish between CSF and abnormalities much easier as compared to other sequences. In this sequence, CSF is attenuated and made darker, but abnormalities remain highlighted.

TABLE 7.1
Statistical features of MRI images

Images	Mean	Standard Deviation	Skewness	Entropy
MRI 1	7.9	44.1	0.00554	0.62
MRI 2	12.5	50.1	0.00657	0.92
MRI 3	40	76	0.01058	3.00
MRI 4	7	40	0.00513	0.44
MRI 5	10	38.25	0.02008	2.07
MRI 6	6.33	29.5	0.01647	1.15

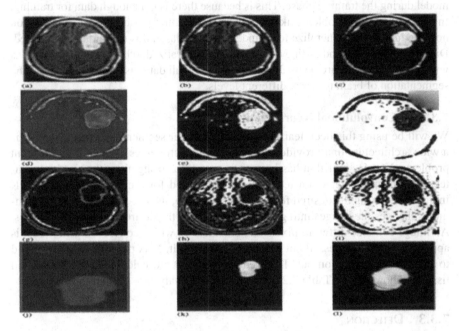

FIGURE 7.5 Brain tumor segmentation.

Moreover, T1 contrast enhanced (T1C) images are also used to identify a more specific type of tumor. The T1C is just like T1-weighted images but with the contrast enhanced. The segmentation of tumor from brain images gives an efficient and accurate result of a series of MRI brain slices combined after preprocessing them. The main objective of preprocessing is to remove all the irrelevant areas such as eyes and skull, remove the homogeneities due to movement of the subject (patient), and remove in homogeneities due to ionizing radiations emitted from the MRI scanner.

7.3.2 Segmentation

The BRATS challenge dataset that we have contains 210 MR images of HGG tumors and 75 MR images of LGG patients. We will be taking random data of 201 MRIs from this dataset for training and testing procedures. First, we will be doing segmentation on MRIs via different algorithms and architectures then we will be performing detection techniques via generative models.

7.3.2.1 Three-Fold Cross-Validation

It is also known as k-fold cross validation technique. It has to be ensured that the models have got most of the patterns from the data correct, de-noised (as we did in preprocessing). The purpose of cross-validation is to define a data set for testing the model during the training phase. This is because there is not enough data for training. In order to limit the problems like overfitting, under fitting, and also get an insight on how the model will generalize to an independent dataset, this technique is preferred. Distribution training and testing data should be generalized; otherwise the predictions will not meet our requirements. It works best on small datasets. Figure 7.4 shows the segmentation of brain tumor at different levels.

7.3.2.2 Convolutional Neural Network (CNN)

We will be using this deep learning algorithm in our segmentation procedure. It is a wide architecture that provides us with different strategies to overcome different problems. YOLO algorithm has been proven to be a strong algorithm in this architecture. An image detection technique will be used for the segmentation of MR images for getting the desired features. Furthermore, its non-max suppression technique changes the images into grids and provide us the desired grids with necrosis. An image contains different pixels and channels on which convolved grid kernel is applied to get a suppressed but comprehensive result. Max pooling will be applied to get the maximum output. Different parameters are calculated for segmented tissue as shown in the Table 7.2 and its graphical analysis as shown in Figure 7.6.

7.3.3 Detection

7.3.3.1 K-Nearest Neighbour

The five crucial steps of the K-NN classification are: determining the k value, calculating the distance between the training samples and the query instance, distances are sorted according to the kth minimal distance, majority class assignment and class determination. This algorithm focuses on classification and regression. The object is mostly classified by the characteristics of its neighbors. Both classification and regression work on a principle of the voting and plurality of the neighbors. This technique also works for feature extraction. Using our dataset, different techniques will be applied on it.

7.3.3.2 Kernel SVM

Kernel SVM works much better than simple support vector machine as it combines different results of SVM and gives one optimal result. Using the techniques for feature extraction, the whole process will be applied. The classification and comparison

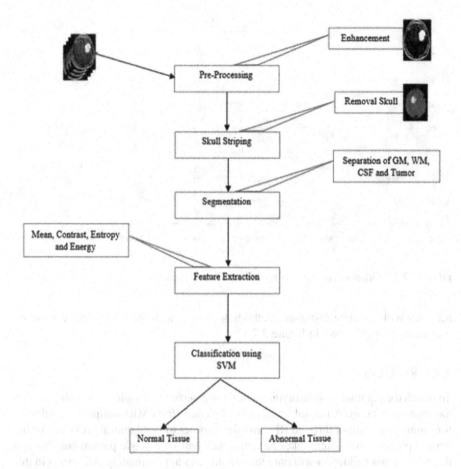

FIGURE 7.6 Flow diagram of segmentation and classification of brain tumor.

TABLE 7.2
Segmented tissues: Parameter results

Images	MSE	PSNR (dB)	SSIM	Dice Score
MRI 1	1.20	59.7	0.8803	0.77
MRI 2	4.90	57.3	0.9700	0.81
MRI 3	5.0	58.5	0.7971	0.89
MRI 4	0.55	69.2	0.9021	0.85
MRI 5	1.80	56.40	0.8940	0.82

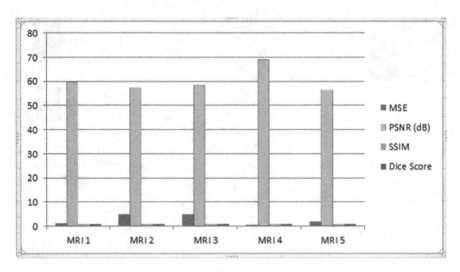

FIGURE 7.7 Graphical analysis of segmented tissue parameters.

accuracy with the state-of-the-art methods are shown in Table 7.3 and corresponding graphical analysis shown in Figure 7.7.

7.4 RESULTS

To match the parameters in arrhythmia order, we performed triple cross-validation on the training data set. An equal number of LGG and HGG MRI samples are selected for training the dataset through RF classifier in order to yield optimal results. For the normal process, the system takes an hour and a half on a single patient but, through three-fold cross validation will only take 15 minutes approximately. All results in this work are obtained by using Python language on two different IDEs: MATLAB and SPYDER. Observations in this work suggested that if the tumor tissue intensities are below the mean intensity of the image, the necrosis tissues are classified as tumorous. YOLO algorithm has also shown us some promising results in the segmentation of the MR images. Using non-max suppression, this algorithm takes less time as compared to three-fold cross validation. Using YOLO algorithm, it eliminates all the normal and non-tumorous parts in the MRI and detects the infectious part of the brain. This methodology is derived from CNN and it could be used as well for the detection of a brain tumor. As we have already discussed before, the structure of a brain can deviate from an average brain, but we cannot declare it a tumor. For detection, we have used generative models as three-fold cross validation gives us promising results, but our approach was to use both models in order to compare the results and as shown in Table 7.3. Accuracy and other parameters have been calculated for the proposed algorithm and compared with the state-of-the-art methods as shown in Table 7.4. It's concluded that the proposed method achieves 90% accuracy. Table 7.4 shows the performance analysis of various parameters with the state-of-the-art comparison and its graphical analysis shown in Figure 7.8.

TABLE 7.3
Classification and comparison accuracy with state-of-the-art methods

Supervised Classifiers	Accuracy (%) without Feature Extraction	Accuracy (%) with Feature Extraction
ANFIS [20]	84.6	90.00
Back Propagation [6]	79.25	84.57
SVM (proposed Classifier)	90.01	95.51
KNN [3]	83.55	87.02

TABLE 7.4
Test images (Abnormal =185, Normal = 100)

Result Parameters	Neuro Fuzzy Inference System (ANFIS) [20]	Back Propagation [6]	SVM (Proposed Classifier)	KNN [3]
True Negative	59	59	59	59
False Negative	14	20	5	16
True Positive	121	108	135	109
False Negative	5	09	4	9
Specificity (%)	81.32	69.67	93.1	79.66
Sensitivity (%)	97.86	98.7	98.61	94.44
Accuracy (%)	89.04	87.43	94.42	86.32

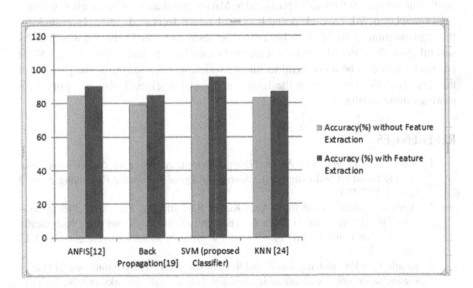

FIGURE 7.8 Graphical analysis of classification and comparison accuracy with state-of-the-art methods.

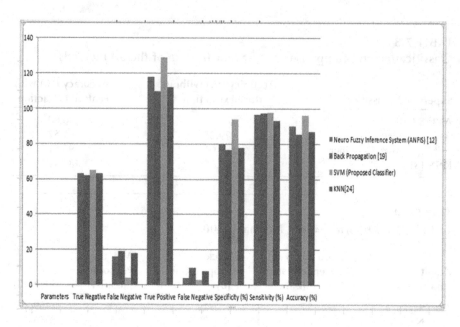

FIGURE 7.9 Performance analysis of various parameters with state-of-the-art comparison.

7.5 CONCLUSION

This chapter contributes to both segmentation and detection of a brain tumor using CNN architecture and different machine learning algorithms. Most of the papers we studied in our research either contributed to MRI segmentation or automation of brain tumor detection. We have proposed a system which works on CNN algorithms for the segmentation of the MRI for obtaining the desired results. Detection was done by several algorithms in order to get the desired as well as optimal results. Kernel SVM has been proven to be a powerful technique which serves and fulfills the purpose of this research. Furthermore, in the future, additional work will also be applied for more accurate results.

REFERENCES

1. Nagalkar, V.J., and S.S. Asole. "Brain tumor detection using digital image processing based on soft computing." *Journal of Signal and Image Processing* 3, no. 3 (2012): 102–105.
2. Bahadure, Nilesh Bhaskarrao, Arun Kumar Ray, and Har Pal Thethi. "Image analysis for MRI based brain tumor detection and feature extraction using biologically inspired BWT and SVM." *International Journal of Biomedical Imaging* 2017 17 (2017): 12.
3. Saouli, Rachida, Mohamed Akil, and Rostom Kachouri. "Fully automatic brain tumor segmentation using end-to-end incremental deep neural networks in MRI images." *Computer Methods and Programs in Biomedicine* 166 (2018): 39–49.

4. Havaei, Mohammad, Axel Davy, David Warde-Farley, Antoine Biard, Aaron Courville, Yoshua Bengio, Chris Pal, Pierre-Marc Jodoin, and Hugo Larochelle. "Brain tumor segmentation with deep neural networks." *Medical Image Analysis* 35 (2017): 18–31.
5. Mohsen, Heba, El-Sayed A. El-Dahshan, El-Sayed M. El-Horbaty, and Abdel-Badeeh M. Salem. "Classification using deep learning neural networks for brain tumors." *Future Computing and Informatics Journal* 3, no. 1 (2018): 68–71.
6. Pereira, Sérgio, Adriano Pinto, Victor Alves, and Carlos A. Silva. "Brain tumor segmentation using convolutional neural networks in MRI images." *IEEE Transactions on Medical Imaging* 35, no. 5 (2016): 1240–1251.
7. Hussain, Saddam, Syed Muhammad Anwar, and Muhammad Majid. "Segmentation of glioma tumors in brain using deep convolutional neural network." *Neurocomputing* 282 (2018): 248–261.
8. Pinto, Adriano, Sérgio Pereira, Deolinda asteiro, and Carlos A. Silva. "Hierarchical brain tumour segmentation using extremely randomized trees." *Pattern Recognition* 82 (2018): 105–117.
9. Anaraki, Amin Kabir, Moosa Ayati, and Foad Kazemi. "Magnetic resonance imaging-based brain tumor grades classification and grading via convolutional neural networks and genetic algorithms." *Biocybernetics and Biomedical Engineering* 39, no. 1 (2019): 63–74.
10. Milletari, Fausto, Seyed-Ahmad Ahmadi, Christine Kroll, Annika Plate, Verena Rozanski, Juliana Maiostre, Johannes Levin et al. "Hough-CNN: deep learning for segmentation of deep brain regions in MRI and ultrasound." *Computer Vision and Image Understanding* 164 (2017): 92–102.
11. Kamnitsas, Konstantinos, Christian Ledig, Virginia F.J. Newcombe, Joanna P. Simpson, Andrew D. Kane, David K. Menon, Daniel Rueckert, and Ben Glocker. "Efficient multi-scale 3D CNN with fully connected CRF for accurate brain lesion segmentation." *Medical Image Analysis* 36 (2017): 61–78.
12. Prastawa, Marcel, Elizabeth Bullitt, Sean Ho, and Guido Gerig. "A brain tumor segmentation framework based on outlier detection." *Medical Image Analysis* 8, no. 3 (2004): 275–283.
13. Zacharaki, Evangelia I., Sumei Wang, Sanjeev Chawla, Dong Soo Yoo, Ronald Wolf, Elias R. Melhem, and Christos Davatzikos. "Classification of brain tumor type and grade using MRI texture and shape in a machine learning scheme." *Magnetic Resonance in Medicine: An Official Journal of the International Society for Magnetic Resonance in Medicine* 62, no. 6 (2009): 1609–1618.
14. Kumar, Sanjeev, Chetna Dabas, and Sunila Godara. "Classification of brain MRI tumor images: a hybrid approach." *Procedia Computer Science* 122 (2017): 510–517.
15. Zotin, Alexander, Konstantin Simonov, Mikhail Kurako, Yousif Hamad, and Svetlana Kirillova. "Edge detection in MRI brain tumor images based on fuzzy C-means clustering." *Procedia Computer Science* 126 (2018): 1261–1270.
16. Abdel-Maksoud, Eman, Mohammed Elmogy, and Rashid Al-Awadi. "Brain tumor segmentation based on a hybrid clustering technique." *Egyptian Informatics Journal* 16, no. 1 (2015): 71–81.
17. Bauer, Stefan, Lutz-P. Nolte, and Mauricio Reyes. "Fully automatic segmentation of brain tumor images using support vector machine classification in combination with hierarchical conditional random field regularization." In *International Conference on Medical Image Computing and Computer-assisted Intervention*, pp. 354–361. Springer, Berlin, Heidelberg, 2011.

18. Cabria, Iván, and Iker Gondra. "MRI segmentation fusion for brain tumor detection." *Information Fusion* 36 (2017): 1–9.
19. Tong, Jijun, Yingjie Zhao, Peng Zhang, Lingyu Chen, and Lurong Jiang. "MRI brain tumor segmentation based on texture features and kernel sparse coding." *Biomedical Signal Processing and Control* 47 (2019): 387–392.
20. Işın, Ali, Cem Direkoğlu, and Melike Şah. "Review of MRI-based brain tumor image segmentation using deep learning methods." *Procedia Computer Science* 102 (2016): 317–324.
21. Rehman, Zaka Ur, Syed S. Naqvi, Tariq M. Khan, Muhammad A. Khan, and Tariq Bashir. "Fully automated multi-parametric brain tumour segmentation using superpixel based classification." *Expert Systems with Applications* 118 (2019): 598–613.
22. Aslam, Asra, Ekram Khan, and M.M. Sufyan Beg. "Improved edge detection algorithm for brain tumor segmentation." *Procedia Computer Science* 58 (2015): 430–437.
23. Amin, Javeria, Muhammad Sharif, Mussarat Yasmin, and Steven Lawrence Fernandes. "Big data analysis for brain tumor detection: Deep convolutional neural networks." *Future Generation Computer Systems* 87 (2018): 290–297.
24. Zikic, Darko, Yani Ioannou, Matthew Brown, and Antonio Criminisi. "Segmentation of brain tumor tissues with convolutional neural networks." Proceedings MICCAI-BRATS 36, no. 2014 (2014): 36–39.
25. Sajjad, Muhammad, Salman Khan, Khan Muhammad, Wanqing Wu, Amin Ullah, and Sung Wook Baik. "Multi-grade brain tumor classification using deep CNN with extensive data augmentation." *Journal of Computational Science* 30 (2019): 174–182.
26. Chen, Shengcong, Changxing Ding, and Minfeng Liu. "Dual-force convolutional neural networks for accurate brain tumor segmentation." *Pattern Recognition* 88 (2019): 90–100.
27. Zhao, Xiaomei, Yihong Wu, Guidong Song, Zhenye Li, Yazhuo Zhang, and Yong Fan. "A deep learning model integrating FCNNs and CRFs for brain tumor segmentation." *Medical Image Analysis* 43 (2018): 98–111.
28. Zhou, Chenhong, Changxing Ding, Xinchao Wang, Zhentai Lu, and Dacheng Tao. "One-pass multi-task networks with cross-task guided attention for brain tumor segmentation." *IEEE Transactions on Image Processing* 29 (2020): 4516–4529.
29. Zhou, Tongxue, Stéphane Canu, Pierre Vera, and Su Ruan. "Brain tumor segmentation with missing modalities via latent multi-source correlation representation." In International Conference on Medical Image Computing and Computer-Assisted Intervention, pp. 533–541. Springer, Cham, 2020.
30. Zhou, T., S. Canu, P. Vera, and S. Ruan. Latent correlation representation learning for brain tumor segmentation with missing MRI modalities. *IEEE Transactions on Image Processing* 30 (2021): 4263–4274. https://doi. org/10.1109/TIP.2021.3070752
31. Zhou, T., S. Ruan, Y. Guo, and S. Canu (2020) A multi-modality fusion network based on attention mechanism for brain tumor segmentation. In: 2020 IEEE 17th International Symposium on Biomedical Imaging (ISBI), pp. 377–380.
32. Almadhoun, Hamza Rafiq, and Samy S. Abu-Naser. "Detection of brain tumor using deep learning." *International Journal of Academic Engineering Research* (IJAER) 6, no. 3 (2022): 29–47.
33. Arif, Muhammad, F. Ajesh, Shermin Shamsudheen, Oana Geman, Diana Izdrui, and Dragos Vicoveanu. "Brain tumor detection and classification by MRI using

biologically inspired orthogonal wavelet transform and deep learning techniques." *Journal of Healthcare Engineering* 2022 4 (2022): 1–18.
34. Sharif, Muhammad Imran, Muhammad Attique Khan, Musaed Alhussein, Khursheed Aurangzeb, and Mudassar Raza. "A decision support system for multimodal brain tumor classification using deep learning." *Complex & Intelligent Systems* 8, no. 4 (2022): 3007–3020.

8 Application of Image Processing in the Detection of Plant Diseases

*Pawan Whig, Nasmin Jiwani, Ketan Gupta,
Shama Kouser, Arun Velu and Ashima Bhatia*

8.1 INTRODUCTION

In today's scenario, farming land is used for additional than just feeding. The Indian economy is heavily reliant on agricultural output. Due to this, in the arena of farming, illness discovery in plants is dangerous. The use of an involuntary disease discovery method can help detect a plant disease in its early stages. For example, little leaf illness is a dangerous illness originating in pine trees in the United States (Whig, Velu, & Naddikatu, 2022).

The pretentious tree grows slowly and dies after six years. It has an impact on Alabama, Georgia, and other shares of the southern United States. In such cases, the initial discovery might remain beneficial (Alkali et al., 2022a).

The current approach for plant illness discovery is through a skilled bare eye remark for the identification and detection of plant diseases. To accomplish this, a huge team of professionals as well as regular plant monitoring is necessary, which is quite expensive when dealing with great farms (Whig, Velu, & Sharma, 2022).

Meanwhile, in some nations, farmers lack the resources or even the skills to get in touch with experts. Therefore, hiring professionals is expensive and time-consuming. One example of the architecture of leaf disease detection systems is given in Figure 8.1. In such cases, the recommended approach is useful for monitoring huge agricultural fields. The automatic identification of illnesses by simply looking at the ciphers on the plant greeneries simplifies and reduces costs.

The identification of phytopathogens by eye requires greater time and accuracy, and it must be done in certain places. Whereas using an automated detection approach will need less work, less time, and will be more accurate (Jupalle et al., 2022). Plants frequently get brown and yellow patches, early and late scorch, and several fungi, viruses, and microbial illnesses. Image analysis is used to measure the affected area of sickness and evaluate the color change of an injured region.

Picture division is the process of unraveling or alliance various elements of a double as shown in Figure 8.2. Picture segmentation may be performed in a variety

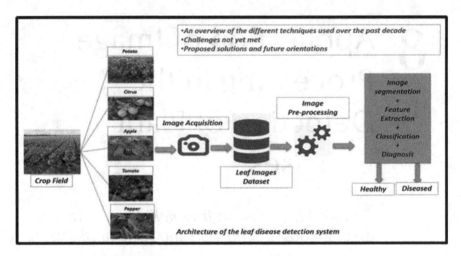

FIGURE 8.1 Architecture of leaf diseases detection system.

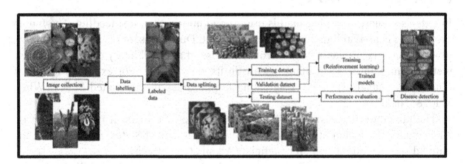

FIGURE 8.2 Picture segmentation process.

of ways, ranging from simple thresholding to complex color image segmentation approaches. Normally, these pieces relate to somewhat that people can readily distinguish and see as independent things. Because processers cannot recognize things intelligently, numerous alternative methods for segmenting photos have been devised. The segmentation technique is based on numerous picture properties (Tomar et al., 2021). This might be color data, picture borders, or a fragment of an image. For color picture segmentation, we employ the genetic algorithm.

For a long time, identifying leaf diseases has been a major issue in agriculture. Plant disease prediction is highly dependent on three factors: host, environment, and pathogens. Plant disease detection systems may be built effectively if their capabilities and the processes that fuel present disease identification systems are understood. However, research in plant pathology shows that plant disease detection is now moving at the speed of light. Startups have begun to develop smartphone applications that utilize image-based algorithms to diagnose plant illness and offer advice on how to properly care for plants, but the algorithms cannot currently assess plants in diverse lighting conditions (Anand et al., 2022). When the environment changes, such as gloomy, overcast, and bright situations, the efficiency of algorithms decreases substantially, calling into doubt the accuracy power of algorithms established thus far.

Even with data augmentation and more diversified training data, supervised learning has failed to improve. Computer vision techniques such as picture classification, segmentation, and object identification have the potential to develop a very precise and accurate system capable of identifying any sort of crop species, but the road ahead is lengthy. Following breakthroughs in deep learning, many articles were published that demonstrated how to train a deep neural network to recognize diverse crop species. A few years back, researchers published a study in which they demonstrated how to train a deep convolutional neuronic net to detect 14 crop classes and 26 illnesses with correctness of 99.35% on the exercise set and 31.4% on the examination set. It was a competitive dataset that had been cleansed in the lab, but in real life, when farmers are faced with this sort of system, a change in environmental circumstances will be a speed breaker in growing healthy crops. Since then, several articles have embraced the approach of utilizing deep convolutional networks to diagnose disease on diverse crop species, whether employing a single crop like tomato or thousands of crops and their species to create cutting-edge plant disease identification findings (Madhu & Whig, 2022).

This chapter provides a complete explanation of artificial neural network learning, demonstrating how backpropagation trains neurons to discriminate between different forms of leaf disease. It is detailed on how to use gradient-based visualization approaches to evaluate multiple activation maps of learned characteristics and then investigate the potential of utilizing a different learning strategy.

8.2 VARIOUS LIMITATIONS UNDER THE IMPACT OF LIGHT

8.2.1 Lighting Difficulties

Images of plant diseases and pests have been gathered for previous research mostly in indoor lightboxes. Although this technique can successfully reduce the impact of outside light to streamline picture processing, it differs significantly from photographs taken in actual natural light. It is simple to produce picture color distortion when above or below this limit since natural light fluctuates extremely animatedly and the variety in which the photographic camera can accept lively light foundations is restricted. Additionally, the apparent features of plant diseases and pests fluctuate significantly owing to variations in view angle and distance during image collection, which presents significant challenges to the visual identification system (Chopra & WHIG, 2022b).

8.2.2 Occlusion Issue

Currently, the majority of researchers purposefully avoid identifying plant diseases and pests in complicated ecosystems. They just pay attention to one background. Instead of taking into account the occlusion issue, they frequently use the technique of directly interjecting the area of care in the composed images. As a result, the practicability and identification accuracy under occlusion are both quite poor. Occlusion issues, such as blade occlusion brought on by vicissitudes in blade carriage, branch occlusion, light obstruction brought on by outside lighting, and varied obstruction brought on by various kinds of blocking, are frequent in actual natural environments (Chopra & Whig, 2022a).

Occlusion is complicated and unpredictable though. We need to improve the basic framework's innovation and optimization, including the development of lightweight network architecture, because basic framework training is challenging and there is still a reliance on hardware device performance. While assuring the accuracy of detection, the investigation of GAN and other elements should be strengthened, and the challenge of perfect exercise should be diminished. GAN offers clear benefits in handling carriage vicissitudes and a disordered environment, but because of its immature design, it is prone to crashes during learning and might lead to unmanageable issues with the model while being trained. To make it simpler to measure the model's quality, we should expand our investigation of network performance (Chopra & Whig, 2022b).

8.2.3 Detection Speed Issue

Deep learning algorithms produce better results than more conventional techniques, but they also have more computational complexity. If the detection accuracy is assured, the model must completely comprehend the image's features and add to its computing burden, which will ultimately result in a slow detection speed that cannot keep up with real-time demands. Usually, less calculation needs to be done to guarantee detection speed. But this will lead to inadequate training and erroneous. So, it is crucial to create an effective procedure that has rapid and accurate discovery (Whig, Velu, & Ready, 2022).

Data labeling, model training, and model inference are the three key components of deep learning-based approaches for detecting plant diseases and pests in agricultural applications. More focus is placed on model inference in real-time agricultural applications. Today, the majority of plant disease and pest detection techniques emphasize precise identification. The efficiency of model inference receives less consideration (Whig, Kouser, Velu, et al., 2022). A deep divisible difficulty construction perfect for plant leaf disease discovery was obtainable by increasing the effectiveness of the model calculation process to accommodate the actual agricultural demands. The training and testing of several models. Reduced MobileNet's classification accuracy was 99.14%; its limits were 29 times smaller than VGG's and six times smaller than MobileNet's.

To enhance production, accurate early diagnosis of plant illnesses is crucial. Because of the tiny size of the cut thing situation, various downsampling operations in the deep eye removal net tend to neglect limited objects in the real early diagnosis of plant diseases and pests. Furthermore, large-scale complex backgrounds may result in more false detection because of the background noise issue in the gathered photos, especially on low-resolution images. The direction of tiny object identification algorithm enhancement is examined in light of the dearth of current algorithms,

Application of Image Processing in Detecting Plant Diseases

and several tactics, including attention mechanisms, are suggested to enhance the effectiveness of small target detection (Whig, Velu, & Nadikattu, 2022).

Resource allocation becomes more logical when attention mechanisms are used. Finding a region of interest rapidly and ignoring irrelevant information is the core function of the attention mechanism. The background noise in a picture may be reduced by applying the weighted sum approach with a weighted coefficient to separate features after learning the characteristics of images of plant diseases and pests (Whig, Velu, & Bhatia, 2022).

8.3 EXPERIMENT DESIGN

This research focused on the visualization of feature detection during the backpropagation process by a deep neural network.

This is accomplished through the use of gradient-based visualization techniques; the methods listed below are used to assess learned features:

1. Vanilla backpropagation
2. Integrated gradients
3. Guided backpropagation
4. Grad-CAM

The photos in this study were obtained from the Plant Village Dataset. It is used to create photos of tomato leaves afflicted with various infections. It is divided into ten classes: nine varieties of tomato leaf illnesses and healthy leaf photos as shown in Figure 8.3. A convolutional neural network has been fine-tuned using such pictures; it gets a three-channel input image of size 224 × 224 and returns a ten-dimensional vector with tomato leaf recognition probability (Alkali et al., 2022a).

The photos are chosen from three tomato leaf disease categories: septoria leaf spot, bacterial spot, and mosaic virus; each disease is caused by a different type of pathogen. Following that, comparisons across all three illness categories are made, and representative maps are constructed to gain geographical information regarding visually interpretable hotspots (Khera et al., 2021). Convolutional neural network has been trained using transfer learning as shown in Figure 8.4, and the One Cycle learning policy is employed for quicker network training using the Fast.ai package.

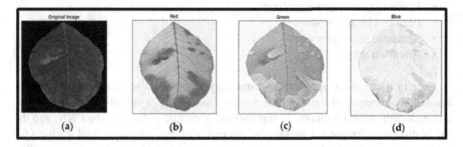

FIGURE 8.3 Vanilla backpropagation.

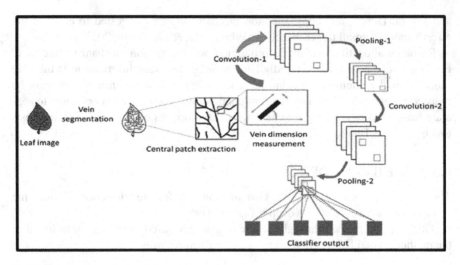

FIGURE 8.4 Convolutional neural network.

Normalized images were created with pixel values ranging from [0.0, to 0.1]. To train the neural network, the ADAM optimization technique is used with the categorical cross-entropy loss measure. Gradient-based visualization is then used to examine and depict the outcomes of the learned feature (Whig & Ahmad, 2014).

8.4 RELATED WORKS

With an anticipated yield of 18,735.91 thousand metric tonnes, tomato is India's most important horticultural crop. Tomato plants have over 7,500 variations and are susceptible to 200 pests and diseases. Aside from that, tomato is taken in a variety of ways, raw or cooked, making them more dangerous to those who consume them. Tomato leaf disease is a huge problem that costs farmers a lot of money and poses a danger to the agriculture industry (Velu & Whig, 2021).

Several strategies have been presented on the subject of Explainable Computer Vision to investigate and interpret what convolutional neural networks have learned. They primarily fall into four visualization method categories:

- Hidden layer output visualization
- Feature visualization
- Semantic dictionary
- Attention map.

Each of these visualization maps causes layer activation within a neural network. Hidden layer output visualization techniques are the most straightforward for visualizing a deep neural network. In this method, a picture is fed into the CNN, and the calculation is interrupted at the layer of interest, with the same methodology used for each layer to extract the learned feature in interpretable form as shown in Figure 8.5.

Application of Image Processing in Detecting Plant Diseases

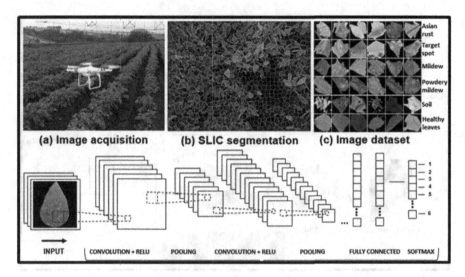

FIGURE 8.5 Classification process using CNN.

Feature visualization techniques are used to display the CNN feature by analyzing the activity of relevant neurons using a gradient ascent strategy. In this method, the neural network receives a picture with random noise, and the gradient of the input image is computed. Gradients are applied to the input image to calculate the mean output of values for the target neuron (Nadikattu et al., 2020).

Attention maps allow us to collect spatial information about the input picture using Semantic Dictionary, which is a mix of feature visualization and intermediate output visualization. While semantic dictionaries help us understand the picture classification process, activation maps help us understand how gradient adjusts the weights of a deep neural network. Gradient-based visualization approaches are used to visualize features and obtain activation maps from networks.

Gradient-based visualization approaches are used to comprehend how backpropagation algorithms train a network that has learned to recognize specific lesions associated with a leaf disease as shown in Figure 8.6. Gradient-based visualization approaches are used to determine which neurons activate inside a trained convolutional neural network when an input picture is identified.

8.4.1 Case Study

An input picture is sent through the network using gradient-based algorithms, and changes in gradient values are computed. Table 8.1 compares photos to compare and appreciate how backpropagation updates the particular levels of the network for leaf disease detection. When a picture is transmitted through the network, various groups of illnesses display distinct activations. These technologies provide us with diverse activation maps that allow us to identify different forms of plant diseases that the network has learned to recognize.

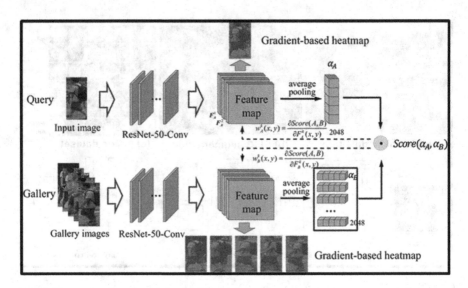

FIGURE 8.6 Gradient-based visualization approaches.

We may use these approaches to analyze spatial information and determine whether parts of a picture are infected with a given virus. The visualization produced by various approaches is summarized in Table 8.1.

The feature learned by the neural network layers is displayed and contrasted using visualization tools. By examining Table 8.1, the sensitivity of gradients has been compared with vanilla backpropagation and integrated gradients; both vanilla backpropagation and integrated gradients indicate activation from backgrounds fired rather than neurons that are closer to lesions in the picture. Both of these strategies are too general. It has been demonstrated that guided backpropagation alone may identify certain diseases and parts of leaf activation that the network has trained to recognize.

Grad-CAM was used to activate a specific activation of class when an input picture about it was sent through the network; nevertheless, it lacked specificity. Grad-CAM is affected by the size of the intermediate output; thus when activation occurs via shallow layers, it reveals lesions more than deeper ones.

The activation maps created by several gradient-based visualization maps of diseased tomato leaf diseases are compared in this study. Deep learning provides state-of-the-art results in plant disease identification, but traditional computer vision techniques also achieve significant accuracy when using the Tree-Based Pipeline Optimization Tool (TPOT). Tree-Based Pipeline uses genetic programming to perform classification by using a plant leaf dataset with significant preprocessing, and it is possible to achieve the same result as given by neural networks. To accomplish illness detection, semi-supervised learning might be used instead of supervised learning. Because real-world data is far more complicated and data scientists are not always able to supply cleansed and labeled datasets, developing unsupervised learning techniques should be prioritized.

Application of Image Processing in Detecting Plant Diseases 233

TABLE 8.1
Gradient-based visualization

Input Image	Grad-CAM	Guided Back-Propagation	Vanilla Back-Propagation	Integrated Gradients

However, because unsupervised learning on a dataset cannot yet be used to achieve the aim, there should be much more potential for developing biological forms of learning. New research was published last year that outlines how traditional forms of backpropagation are physiologically impossible.

This case study examines a semi-supervised learning technique that employs global inhibition in hidden layers by learning early feature detectors unsupervised. Instead of supervised learning with backpropagation, it employs a unique learning rule based on Hebb's theory that synapse strength should be local – that is, synapse strength should only be affected by the actions of pre- and post-synaptic neurons. Both of these techniques can classify tomato leaf diseases with comparable accuracy to deep neural networks.

8.5 CHALLENGES

8.5.1 Problem with Small Dataset Sizes

Deep learning techniques are currently widely employed in many computer vision applications, and the identification of plant diseases and pests is typically considered to be a specialized application in the field of agriculture. There are not enough samples of agricultural plant diseases and pests. Self-collected data sets are laboriously labeled and smaller in size than open standard library. In actuality the image data set of plan illness are of low occurrence hence the collecting charges are also high. In reality, there are now three possible solutions to the small sample problem. The problem of tiny samples is the most pressing issue facing the identification of plant diseases and pests, as opposed to the more than 14 million sample data in ImageNet datasets.

8.5.2 Data Amplification, Synthesis, and Production

A vital step in developing deep learning models is data amplification. The detection of plant diseases and pests can be significantly enhanced by a well-designed data amplification method. The most popular technique for expanding plant disease and pest images is to use the original plant illnesses and pest samples as a starting point to obtain additional examples using image processing processes including reflecting and so on. Additionally, to enrich small datasets.

8.5.3 Transfer Learning Optimization

Transfer learning involves transferring information from specialized fields with sparse quantities of data to general huge datasets. Transfer learning can start with a training model using a comparable known dataset while creating a model for freshly obtained unlabeled samples. It may be used to identify localized plant diseases and pests after tweaking components or adjusting parameters, which can lower the price of perfect exercise and allow the difficult neural net to adapt to tiny example data.

8.5.4 Design of a Reasonable Network Topology

By building an acceptable network topology, the sample needs may be considerably decreased by merging three color components. A channel TCCNN component is made up of three RGB color pictures of the leaf disease. An enhanced CNN approach for detecting grape leaf diseases was described by B. Liu et al. 2000. To prevent overfitting and minimize the number of parameters, the model employed a depth-separable convolution rather than a conventional convolution.

8.6 CONCLUSION

Deep learning-based approaches for detecting plant illnesses and pests integrate them into an end-to-end process for feature extraction that has a lot of growth potential. In contrast, conventional image processing techniques handle jobs like detecting pests and plant diseases in a series of stages and linkages. Even though the expertise for identifying plant pests and diseases has been migrating from scientific work to agricultural uses, it is still some time away from being fully developed for use in the real world of nature, and there are still some issues that need to be resolved.

This work conducts a thorough examination of visible layers of features learned using the backpropagation approach. Layers are shown in the experimental findings using gradient-based visualization approaches such as Grad-CAM, guided backpropagation, vanilla backpropagation, and integrated gradients. Attention maps have been developed to comprehend what region of the input image indicates activation of neurons inside the network, and detection of particular lesions is represented through them. In practice, visualization of each layer provides an interpretation of how a neural network learns to identify different diseases by using gradient-based methods. This study analyzes the process of backpropagation by visualizing the weight updates of the gradient descent optimization process and evaluates how the network learns to identify tomato leaf diseases. As a result, a picture of diseased plants by various types of pathogens is sent through the network, and representative maps of the layers are formed. Grad-CAM is the most descriptive way to create attention maps in this article. It is also the most straightforward and cost-effective technique for visualizing layers.

REFERENCES

Alkali, Y., Routray, I., and Whig, P. (2022a). Strategy for reliable, efficient, and secure IoT using artificial intelligence. *IUP Journal of Computer Sciences*, 16(2), 1–9.

Anand, M., Velu, A., and Whig, P. (2022). Prediction of loan behaviour with machine learning models for secure banking. *Journal of Computer Science and Engineering* (JCSE), 3(1), 1–13.

Chopra, G., and Whig, P. (2022a). Smart agriculture system using AI. *International Journal of Sustainable Development in Computing Science*, 4(1).

Chopra, G., and Whig, P. (2022b). A clustering approach based on support vectors. *International Journal of Machine Learning for Sustainable Development*, 4(1), 21–30.

Jupalle, H., Kouser, S., Bhatia, A. B., Alam, N., Nadikattu, R. R., and Whig, P. (2022). Automation of human behaviors and their prediction using machine learning. *Microsystem Technologies*, 28, 1–9.

Khera, Y., Whig, P., and Velu, A. (2021). Efficient effective and secured electronic billing system using AI. *Vivekananda Journal of Research*, 10, 53–60.

Krizhevsky, A., Sutskever, I., and Hinton, G. E. (2012). Imagenet classification with deep convolutional neural networks, in *Advances in Neural Information Processing Systems*, eds. F. Pereira, C. J. C. Burges, L. Bottou, and K. Q. Weinberger. Curran Associates, Inc., pp. 1097–1105.

LeCun, Y., Bengio, Y., and Hinton, G. (2015). Deep learning. *Nature* 521, 436–444. doi: 10.1038/nature14539

Liu, B., Ding, Z., Tian, L., He, D., and Hongyan Wang, S. L. (2000). Grape leaf disease identification using improved deep convolutional neural networks. In Frontiers in Plant Science 11, article 751.

Lowe, D. G. (2004). Distinctive image features from scale-invariant key points. *International Journal of Computer Vision* 60, 91–110. doi: 10.1023/B:VISI.0000029664.99615.94

Madhu, M., and Whig, P. (2022). A survey of machine learning and its applications. *International Journal of Machine Learning for Sustainable Development*, 4(1), 11–20.

Mokhtar, U., Ali, M. A., Hassanien, A. E., and Hefny, H. (2015). Identifying two of tomatoes leaf viruses using support vector machine, in *Information Systems Design and Intelligent Applications*, eds J. K. Mandal, S. C. Satapathy, M. K. Sanyal, P. P. Sarkar, and A. Mukhopadhyay, Springer, pp. 771–782.

Nadikattu, R. R., Mohammad, S. M., and Whig, P. (2020). Novel economical social distancing smart device for COVID-19. International Journal of Electrical Engineering and Technology (IJEET), 11(4), 204–217.

Russakovsky, O., Deng, J., Su, H., Krause, J., Satheesh, S., Ma, S., et al. (2015). ImageNet large-scale visual recognition challenge. *International Journal of Computer Vision* 115, 211–252. doi: 10.1007/s11263-015-0816-y

Sankaran, S., Mishra, A., Maja, J. M., and Ehsani, R. (2011). Visible-near infrared spectroscopy for detection of huanglongbing in citrus orchards. *Computer Electronics and Agriculture* 77, 127–134. doi: 10.1016/j.compag.2011.03.004

Szegedy, C., Liu, W., Jia, Y., Sermanet, P., Reed, S., Anguelov, D., et al. (2015). Going deeper with convolutions, in Proceedings of the IEEE Conference on Computer Vision and Pattern Recognition.

Tai, A. P., Martin, M. V., and Heald, C. L. (2014). Threat to future global food security from climate change and ozone air pollution. *Nature and Climate Change* 4, 817–821. doi: 10.1038/nclimate2317

Tomar, U., Chakroborty, N., Sharma, H., and Whig, P. (2021). AI-based smart agriculture system. *Transactions on Latest Trends in Artificial Intelligence*, 2(2).

Velu, A., and Whig, P. (2021). Protect personal privacy and wasting time using nlp: A comparative approach using AI. *Vivekananda Journal of Research*, 10, 42–52.

Whig, P., and Ahmad, S. N. (2014). Simulation of a linear dynamic macro model of the photocatalytic sensor in SPICE. *COMPEL The International Journal for Computation and Mathematics in Electrical and Electronic Engineering*, 33(1/2), 611–629.

Whig, P., Kouser, S., Velu, A., & Nadikattu, R. R. (2022). Fog-IoT-assisted-based smart agriculture application. In *Demystifying Federated Learning for Blockchain and Industrial Internet of Things* (pp. 74–93). IGI Global. www.igi-global.com/about/

Whig, P., Velu, A., and Bhatia, A. B. (2022). Protect nature and reduce the carbon footprint with an application of blockchain for IoT. In *Demystifying Federated Learning for Blockchain and Industrial Internet of Things* (pp. 123–142). IGI Global.

Whig, P., Velu, A., and Ready, R. (2022). Demystifying federated learning in artificial intelligence with human-computer interaction. In *Demystifying Federated Learning for Blockchain and Industrial Internet of Things* (pp. 94–122). IGI Global.

Whig, P., Velu, A., and Sharma, P. (2022). Demystifying federated learning for blockchain: A case study. In *Demystifying Federated Learning for Blockchain and Industrial Internet of Things* (pp. 143–165). IGI Global.

Whig, P., Velu, A., and Naddikatu, R. R. (2022). The Economic impact of AI-enabled blockchain in 6G-based industry. In *AI and Blockchain Technology in 6G Wireless Network* (pp. 205–224). Springer, Singapore.

Whig, P., Velu, A., and Nadikattu, R. R. (2022). Blockchain platform to resolve security issues in IoT and smart networks. In *AI-Enabled Agile Internet of Things for Sustainable FinTech Ecosystems* (pp. 46–65). IGI Global.

APPENDIX: SOURCE CODE

```
from fastai.imports import *
from fastai.transforms import *
from fastai.conv_learner import *
from fastai.model import *
from fastai.dataset import *
from fastai.sgdr import *
from fastai.plots import *


PATH = "/home/"
sz = 224
arch=resnet18
bs=64
label_csv = f'train.csv'
n = len(list(open(label_csv))) - 1 # header is not counted (-1)
val_idxs = get_cv_idxs(n) # random 20% data for validation set



tfms = tfms_from_model(arch, sz, aug_tfms=transforms_side_on, max_zoom=1.1)
data = ImageClassifierData.from_csv(PATH, 'images', f'train.csv',
                    val_idxs=val_idxs, tfms=tfms, bs=bs)
learn = ConvLearner.pretrained(resnet18, data, precompute=True, opt_fn=optim.Adam, ps=0.5)

learn.fit(1e-3, 4, cycle_len=1, cycle_mult=2)
lrs=np.array([1e-5,1e-4,1e-3])
learn.precompute=False

learn.unfreeze()
lrf=learn.lr_find(lrs/1e3)
learn.sched.plot()
lrs=np.array([1e-5,1e-4,1e-3])
learn.fit(lrs, 4, cycle_len=1, cycle_mult=2)

log_preds, y = learn.TTA()
probs = np.mean(np.exp(log_preds),0)
accuracy_np(probs, y), metrics.log_loss(y, probs)
```

1 train.py

```python
# contains helper functions for data preprocessing and analysis

import os
import copy
import numpy as np
from PIL import Image
import matplotlib.cm as mpl_color_map

import torch
from torch.autograd import Variable
from torchvision import models

def convert2grayscale(img_as_arr):
    """
    Converts 3d image to grayscale
    Args:
        img_as_arr (numpy arr): RGB image with shape (D,W,H)
    returns:
        grayscale_img (numpy_arr): Grayscale image with shape (1,W,D)
    """
    grayscale_img = np.sum(np.abs(img_as_arr), axis=0)
    img_max = np.percentile(grayscale_img, 99)
    img_min = np.min(grayscale_img)
    grayscale_img = (np.clip((grayscale_img - img_min) / (img_max - img_min), 0, 1))
    grayscale_img = np.expand_dims(grayscale_img, axis=0)
    return grayscale_img

def save_gradients_images(gradients, file_name):
    """
    Exports the original gradients image
    Args:
        gradients (np arr): Numpy array of the gradients with shape (3, 224, 224)
        file_name (str): File name to be exported
    """

    """"""
    if not os.path.exists('results'):
        os.makedirs('results')
    # Normalize
    gradients = gradients - gradients.min()
    gradients /= gradients.max()
    # Save image
    path_to_file = os.path.join('results', file_name + '.jpg')
    save_image(gradients, path_to_file)

def save_class_activation_images(org_img, activation_map, file_name):
    """
    Saves cam activation map and activation map on the original image
```

2 utils.py

Application of Image Processing in Detecting Plant Diseases

```
guided.py
# contains guided gradient back propagation functions

import torch
from torch.nn import ReLU

class GuidedBackprop():
    """
    Produces gradients generated with guided back propagation from the given image
    """
    def __init__(self, model):
        self.model = model
        self.gradients = None
        self.forward_relu_outputs = []
        # Put model in evaluation mode
        self.model.eval()
        self.update_relus()
        self.hook_layers()

    def hook_layers(self):
        def hook_function(module, grad_in, grad_out):
            self.gradients = grad_in[0]
        # Register hook to the first layer
        first_layer = list(self.model.features._modules.items())[0][1]
        first_layer.register_backward_hook(hook_function)

    def update_relus(self):
        """
        Updates relu activation functions so that
            1- stores output in forward pass
            2- imputes zero for gradient values that are less than zero
        """
        def relu_backward_hook_function(module, grad_in, grad_out):
            """
            If there is a negative gradient, change it to zero
            """
            # Get last forward output
            corresponding_forward_output = self.forward_relu_outputs[-1]
            corresponding_forward_output[corresponding_forward_output > 0] = 1
            modified_grad_out = corresponding_forward_output * torch.clamp(grad_in[0], min=0.0)
            del self.forward_relu_outputs[-1]  # Remove last forward output
            return (modified_grad_out,)

        def relu_forward_hook_function(module, ten_in, ten_out):
```

3 vanilla.py

```python
# contains functions to save output of class activation maps

from PIL import Image
import numpy as np
import torch

class CamExtractor():
    """
    Extracts cam features from the model
    """
    def __init__(self, model, target_layer):
        self.model = model
        self.target_layer = target_layer
        self.gradients = None

    def save_gradient(self, grad):
        self.gradients = grad

    def forward_pass_on_convolutions(self, x):
        """
        Does a forward pass on convolutions, hooks the function at given layer
        """
        conv_output = None
        for module_pos, module in self.model.features._modules.items():
            x = module(x)  # Forward
            if int(module_pos) == self.target_layer:
                x.register_hook(self.save_gradient)
                conv_output = x  # Save the convolution output on that layer
        return conv_output, x

    def forward_pass(self, x):
        """
        Does a full forward pass on the model
        """
        # Forward pass on the convolutions
        conv_output, x = self.forward_pass_on_convolutions(x)
        x = x.view(x.size(0), -1)  # Flatten
        # Forward pass on the classifier
        x = self.model.classifier(x)
        return conv_output, x

class GradCam():
    """
    Produces class activation map
```

4 gradcam.py

```python
# contains functions to save the activation of layers performed through integrated gradient based
# visualization

import torch
import numpy as np


class IntegratedGradients():
    """
    Produces gradients generated with integrated gradients from the image
    """
    def __init__(self, model):
        self.model = model
        self.gradients = None
        # Put model in evaluation mode
        self.model.eval()
        # Hook the first layer to get the gradient
        self.hook_layers()

    def hook_layers(self):
        def hook_function(module, grad_in, grad_out):
            self.gradients = grad_in[0]

        # Register hook to the first layer
        first_layer = list(self.model.features._modules.items())[0][1]
        first_layer.register_backward_hook(hook_function)

    def generate_images_on_linear_path(self, input_image, steps):
        # Generate uniform numbers between 0 and steps
        step_list = np.arange(steps+1)/steps
        # Generate scaled xbar images
        xbar_list = [input_image*step for step in step_list]
        return xbar_list

    def generate_gradients(self, input_image, target_class):
        # Forward
        model_output = self.model(input_image)
        # Zero grads
        self.model.zero_grad()
        # Target for backprop
        one_hot_output = torch.FloatTensor(1, model_output.size()[-1]).zero_()
        one_hot_output[0][target_class] = 1
        # Backward pass
        model_output.backward(gradient=one_hot_output)
```

5 integrated_cam.py

9 Preprocessing Sparse and Commonly Evolving Standardised Health Records

C. D. Divya, A. B. Rajendra, and Soundarya Bidare Chandre Gowda

9.1 INTRODUCTION

A person's medical history is recorded in their medical file. Hospitals and doctor's offices frequently employ electronic health. Digital health records for a patient are kept in an electronic health record (EHR)[1]. The terms "medical record," "health record," and "medical chart" are occasionally used interchangeably to describe the methodical documentation of a patient's health record[2] and treatment throughout time under the supervision of an individual health care source [3]. Observations, the management of medicines and therapies, orders for the administration of medications and treatments, test outcomes, x-rays, details, etc. are just a few of the "notes" that healthcare professionals have entered throughout time to create a medical record[4]. Professionals in the medical field and other carers are necessary to keep thorough and accurate medical records. Medical record keeping is required of healthcare professionals and is often enforced as a condition of licensure or certification[5]. The condition of a patient is recorded in their records over time. They must be precise and clear to communicate with patients and other healthcare professionals effectively. The complete fulfilment of a patient's estimated needs is safeguarded by offering accurate medical records[6]. Each medical record must have sufficient specific information to allow for patient identification, diagnosis confirmation, justification of treatment plan, documentation of treatment progress and results, and support of provider continuity of care[7]. The patient's identification details, medical examination results, and health history are all included in the medical record. Additionally, the patient's current and former prescriptions are listed in the medical record. Comprehensiveness, accessibility, interoperability, confidentiality, accountability, and flexibility are traits of an ideal electronic medical records system. Informed care can be given since health care professionals can learn about a patient's medical history through their medical record[8] The medical record acts as the main hub for organising patient care and keeping track of communications between patients, health treatment providers, and other professionals involved in the patient's care. The documentation of conformity

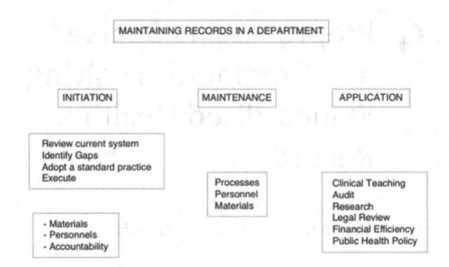

FIGURE 9.1 Maintaining medical records: An overview.

with institutional, professional, or governmental regulation is a function of the medical history that is increasingly important.

Admission documents, on-maintenance notes, improvement notes, preoperative notes, operation documents, postoperative documents, procedure documents, delivery, postpartum and discharge documents can all be found in the standard medical history for inpatient treatment[9]

A patient can share their medical records with other healthcare providers and systems thanks to the combination of several of the capabilities with portability in personal health records [10]. When used in conjunction with genome-wide association studies, electronic medical records can be used to quantify illness problems, like the number of fatalities caused by antimicrobial struggle, or else to determine the effects, contributing components, and contributors to certain diseases [9–[11]. Electronic medical documents may be made accessible for such purposes in strongly anonymised [12] procedures to safeguard patients' confidentiality [12, 14–16] (Figure 9.1).

9.2 LITERATURE SURVEY

In the outpatient departments of the medical centres, the doctors, nurses, and health information management officers are directly involved in the care of the patients. This study has demonstrated that a lack of teamwork and the absence of electronic health record systems are causes of the low patient satisfaction in the chosen medical centre and also lead to lengthy wait times for patients at the university health facilities. According to the current body of research, the study's findings support the need for adequate staff training to enable effective techniques of health information management and to raise patient satisfaction by fostering closer ties with healthcare professionals[13]. To keep accurate health records and improve patient satisfaction with the care they received while hospitalised, the study also made obvious the need for more qualified staff in health information management. The study came to the conclusion that proper handling and filing of patient medical records is crucial to preventing misfiling and loss of patient case files, which could result in extensive information wanted to be able to recognise the patient, show the analysis, defend the progression of treatment, maintain the progress report, and so forth wait times at university medical centres.

Sociodemographic characteristics such as age, prosperity index, place, qualification, employment, marital status, and social position have been shown to be strongly related to the use of Absolute Neutrophil Count (ANC) [14, —15-17]. For instance, Fagbamigbe and Idemudia's cross-sectional study [18] in Nigeria revealed a five-fold rise in ANC usage among women in the richest quintile. According to one of the study, poor women residing in northern Nigeria had a significantly higher risk of not obtaining ANC [19]. The use of ANC is also influenced by other aspects, including insufficient funding, the accessibility of qualified healthcare professionals, especially in rural regions, the gap in ANC facilities, and insufficient health services [20, 21]. Misaligned communication between formal and informal healthcare practitioners is another factor that contributes to poor ANC usage, as does unprofessional behaviour such disrespecting patients' privacy, confidentiality, and traditional beliefs [22 23]. The underutilisation of ANC and the country's poor health outcomes, however, are not caused by one single problem in the country's health care system. Rather, they are the product of numerous problems. A terribly low 0.381 physicians per 1,000 inhabitants is the ratio of health care providers in the nation, as an example. Hospital beds are also in short supply; there are only 0.5 hospital beds for every 1,000 people [24]. Furthermore, inadequate or nonexistent technology health tools hinder the delivery of and access to care. According to the research, Nigeria has subpar methods for managing patient health data, which is largely because these methods have been neglected for a long time, receive insufficient financing, have high wait times at medical facilities, and are not properly stored or accessible [25]. These problems do have an impact on the use of healthcare, which therefore affects adoption of ANC. There is a knowledge gap on the spatial patterns associated with ANC usage, even though numerous research has established the factors of ANC utilisation in Nigeria. The spatial analysis offers a thorough comprehension of demographic characteristics and their impact on the usage of ANC on the environment of health services. This provides a clearer and better grasp of where and what is happening in the research region and aids in solving difficult location-oriented challenges. It aids in comprehending location qualities and their connections to one another. Making decisions is enhanced by spatial analysis [26]. Examining the multilevel influences and spatial supply of ANC usage in Nigeria is crucial to reducing the gap since the country still falls short of the number of ANC visits recommended by the World Health Organization.

9.3 FORMAT OF MEDICAL RECORDS

One of the following formats – Source Oriented Medical Record (SOMR), Problem Oriented Medical Record (POMR), or Integrated Medical Record (IMR) may be used to record a patient's medical history IMR.

9.3.1 SOMR

It is the standard method of recording medical history. Medicinal data is arranged chronologically based on the documentation's source. Its benefits include: it is simple to make and find. It is simple to keep up. It is easy to locate a source's information.

It is challenging and time-consuming to obtain a complete clinical image of a patient.

In the department of medical records, it adds numerous new parts and sub-sections.

For instance, if a nurse documents medical data, preserved under the nursing department, under the laboratory section for the laboratory test, and comes in the radiology section for radiologic test such as x-ray.

9.3.2 POMR

Dr. Lawrence Weed introduced it in the 1960s. It is organised based on every patient's issue or sickness and any relevant medical background. Each problem in this system has a specific number assigned to it, and the problems are primarily arranged in reverse chronological order. There are four sections to it: a database of knowledge, the gathering of information; issues listed: making a list of all the issues; initial strategy formulation of a treatment plan for each issue; a SOAP (subjective, objective, assessment, and plan) note for every issue.

Demerits: Making a fresh report takes a lot of time. It takes some initial training to understand the organisational structure before creating and filing POMR. Information on medicine that relates to multiple issues is repeated.

9.3.3 IMR

It incorporates information from every source that is accessible. Either chronological order or reverse chronological order can be used.

Benefits: Report filing takes less time than before. All instances of a particular diagnosis and therapy are grouped together in this for easy reference.

Merits: It takes time and is difficult to compare information on the same topic. It takes a lot of time and effort to retrieve the relevant information.

9.4 MEDICAL RECORD TYPES

In the modern healthcare system, there are three types of medical records: paper-based, electronic, and mixed. Paper-based medical records are those that are preserved on

TABLE 9.1
Merits of different forms of medical records

PMR	EMR	HMR
Simple	Easily accessible	Nice option to convert from PMR to digital records
No need of technical training	Enhanced security	Alternative to hospitals
Readily available	Reduces administrative costs	

TABLE 9.2
Demerits of different forms of medical records

PMR	EMR	HMR
Requires large volume of storage space, should also be protected from germs.	Might be lost due to system crashes	Accessibility is difficult
Can easily be stolen	Training is needed for the staff to handle this type	Involves excess staff to maintain both manual and electronic records
Illegible hand written records may be hard to decipher	Lack of standardisation makes data exchange difficult	
Huge cost	Huge cost to implement and maintain	

paper. Medical records that are preserved electronically or digitally are referred to as electronic medical records. Medical records that are partially maintained on paper, partially in digital or electronic format are referred to as hybrid records (Tables 9.1 and 9.2).

9.4.1 Ownership of Medical Records

The doctor or hospital is typically the rightful owner of the patient's medical documents, and it is their duty to safeguard that data and uphold patient privacy at all costs. In India, on the other hand, patients retain ownership of their medical records, and they always remain with them. (Government-funded hospitals are an exception.) The patient has all authorised right to ask for a duplicate of the medical documents, to gain access to the medical data as needed, regardless of whether patient is the only owner of the medical data or if they are kept by the hospital.

9.4.2 Raw Medical Data

Protected health information (PHI) is private and will not be disclosed; as a result, it must be de-identified before it can be utilised in research. The technique of de-identification is used to stop a person's individuality from being linked to data. The 18 personal identifiers listed are the simplest approach to de-identify someone. The data is not considered PHI and referred to as basic medical data after de-identification.

Uses of the raw medical data: Governmental organisations and scientific researchers utilise it to create numerous statistical reports, including those on the illness and death rate, residents census, malnourishment index, etc. It is employed by health researchers to identify most effective technique or treatment for a condition. The most efficient and cheap treatments for a given condition should be identified and communicated to the medical community. This, coupled with improved governance and transparency, is thought to help curtail or put an end to cut- or kickback-type practices.

9.4.3 SIGNIFICANCE OF MEDICAL HISTORIES

Medical documents are a collection of information which will be inferred as instructional aids, a foundation for invoicing, connections to ensure continuousness of care throughout follow-ahead, whether in identical or a dissimilar organisation by similar or different doctor. They are essential for enabling proper delivery of healthcare services. Medical records that are properly maintained aid in efficient operation and lower the possibility of human mistake. They are necessary for inspection and research, making them indispensable. They offer clear insight into what happened during earlier visits, which is especially helpful in the developing nations where most of the patients are underprivileged and sizeable percentage of them are uneducated. Medical records that are accurate facilitate simple insurance entitlement or Mediclaim payments. In medicolegal cases, serves as legitimate documented evidence and must be submitted in court when needed. For the patient and the doctor to obtain and give the patient current and ongoing care, a properly maintained medical record is necessary. It is the only piece of documentation the doctor has to support the appropriateness of the patient's care and refute any claims of malpractice. Additionally, it will benefit people who have been the victims of medical malpractice.

9.4.4 COMPONENTS OF A MEDICAL RECORD

- Patient demographic data such as age, sex, nationality, etc.
- Patient demographics include individual information like given name, birth date, address along with insurance facts. Patient demographics make easier health billing, increase the level of healthcare, improve communication, help cultural proficiency. Asking the proper questions, sticking to the laws that are appropriate, and using health related software are required for correctly collecting and documenting patient information [2].
- Social screenings, such as their line of work: it's critical to obtain the data for additional processing.
- Information regarding their genetics: Genetics is the study of genes, genetic diversity, and inheritance in living things. Since heredity is vital to how organisms evolve, it is a crucial subject of biology.

Standardised Health Records

- Current diagnosis and medical history: Information gathered about a patient may be used in any way to direct and oversee care. It is customary to inquire about a patient's medical history when interacting with them for the first time; however, on subsequent visits, this information may only need to be reviewed and possibly updated to reflect any changes. Finding out about important chronic diseases and other prior disease states that may not have been treated but may have had an effect on the patient's health in the long term can be done by getting their medical history. Medicines list: It is crucial to be aware of previous medicine administration.
- List of vaccinations the patient has received.
- Lab test results.
- Diagnostics.
- All their allergies and illnesses so far (see Table 9.3 and Figures 9.2 and 9.3).

TABLE 9.3
Some of the sociodemographic characteristics

Parameters
Gender
Age
Marital Status

Medical history (also known as history and physical, or H&P)
- Patient demographics
- Chief complaint (CC)
- History of present illness (HPI)
- Past medical history (PMH)
- Family history (FH)
- Social history (SH)
- Allergies
- Medication history
- Review of systems (ROS)
- Physical examination (PE)

Laboratory test results
Diagnostic test results
Problem list
Clinical notes
- Progress notes
- Consultation notes
- Off-service notes/transfer notes
- Discharge summary

Treatment notes
- Medication orders
- Surgical procedure documentation
- Radiation treatments
- Notes from ancillary practitioners

FIGURE 9.2 Components of a patient's medical record.

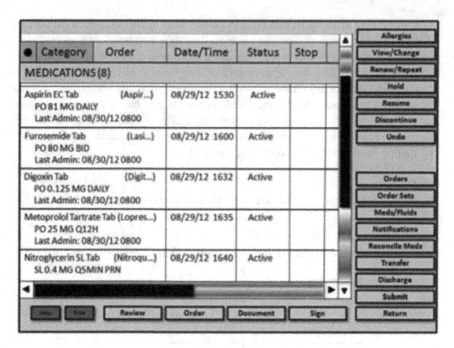

FIGURE 9.3 Example of a computerised prescriber order entry system.

9.4.5 CLASSIFICATION OF MEDICAL HISTORIES

Four significant sections of medical records are listed in the WHO Medical Records manual, and they are as follows:
Demographic and socioeconomic data are administrative.
Legal: Consent is an example.

- Money-related.
- Clinical: whether inpatient or outpatient; elective or emergency, with pertinent medical information

Inpatient records may take the following forms:
The patient's presenting complaints, the length and details of their symptoms, and other pertinent information are included on the history sheet/emergency room admission record, description of their signs, a preliminary diagnosis, a list of any previous and requested investigations, as well as a treatment plan.

Progress sheets: These document the clinical progress of the inpatient while they are hospitalised, as well as the parameters tracked, and interventions performed. It is being recorded in the "SOAP" format per our standard clinical procedure (Figure 9.4).

Standardised Health Records

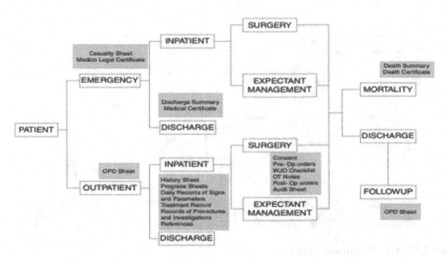

FIGURE 9.4 Records classification.

9.4.6 CLASSIFICATION OF INPATIENT AND OUTPATIENT RECORD

Operative and Postoperative Reports: The thorough operative decisions and phases of process are crucial parts of the record of surgical patients. Every patient should follow an organised template that contains the preoperative diagnosis, the operation's indications, the findings, the surgery (in numbered successive steps), and the postoperative instructions.

References: These serve as a crucial intermediary for all-encompassing patient treatment. Coordinated care is essential, as are clear and concise communications, chronological documentation of the information shared, and following recommendations.

9.4.7 TRADITIONAL SYSTEM

Healthcare analytics design theory and its evaluation receive minimal assistance from conventional system development and prototyping. Common problems include knowledge enhancement, lack of relevance, and the expression of reusable design ideas. By expressing domain-specific concepts or internal practices, daily symptom record (DSR) techniques improve the accuracy and precision of analytics solutions. The outcomes are then used to develop new design expertise for creating and assessing future solutions. While focusing on the IT artefact, design science studies place a significant emphasis on relevance in the application domain. Such efforts have made design research a respectable technique for doing IS research, building on Simon's conceptualisation.

As a cutting-edge methodology, DSR can be useful for the development of certain IS object innovations, including ruling support systems. Agile software development methods that have become the norm for creating analytics applications in the

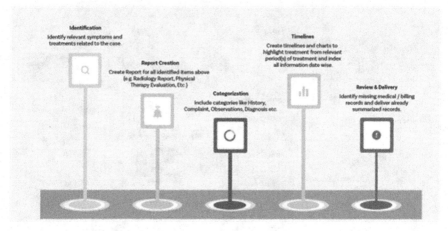

FIGURE 9.5 Preprocessing of data.

healthcare sector. This methodology supports effective means of conducting cooperation and designing analytics solutions. The time typically allotted for an exploration data science development appears to conflict directly with the normal agile development cycle, even though agile must revise to effectively accommodate the hybrid growth field. For their practical stages in eliciting data analytics needs as well as for specifying functional necessities for leveraging information to better company and medical outcomes inside healthcare groups.

9.4.8 MEDICAL SUMMARY PROCESS

Medical data classification (MDC), which strives to raise the standard of healthcare, is the process of learning classification models from medical datasets. Classification of medical data can be used to make diagnoses and forecast outcomes. Medical data have characteristics, such as noise brought on by systematic and human mistakes, missing values, and even sparsity. Quality of the mining results is significantly impacted by the quality of the data. To eliminate or at least lessen some of the issues related to medical data, preparation procedures must be carried out (Figure 9.5).

9.5 REVIEW OF THE METHODS ADOPTED

9.5.1 ANTMINER ALGORITHM

A majority class-related default rule and a sequential-covering approach are used in the construction of the AntMiner. In essence, rule induction focuses on classes other than the dominant class. This technique is helpful in the classification of medical data because the majority of class instances are often the unfavourable circumstances, which we don't care about as much. The sequential-covering method helps with handling large datasets by gradually reducing the size of the training set by removing

Standardised Health Records

examples that have already been covered by induced rules. The AntMiner algorithm is unable to handle instances with missing values. Deleting these instances from the dataset is therefore the first step. To reduce the size of the solution space, the number of characteristics is limited to only one default value.

Minimal-cost, low-power electronics are simple to buy and operate. Although some characteristics, such as temperature, blood pressure, can be accurately recorded, developers are attempting to target an increasing number of features. Digital health software and devices are certified by the Food and Drug Administration (FDA) and European Medicines Agency (EMA). Most products on the market do not meet the minimal requirements for accreditation and certification. Some of these have been widely utilised in highly polluted cities as air quality monitoring tools. However, due to the extremely poor data quality produced by home devices, no medical organisation advises doing so; instead, only using data from authorised official stations.

9.5.2 IoT Programmes for e-Health Purposes

Thinger.io: An alternative is open source IoT platform. Though Thinger.io is still a relative newcomer to IoT environment, it has already been heavily utilised among numerous research plans [25] and teaching. It provides a ready-to-use cloud service for tethering devices to the Internet to do any remote sensing or actuation over the Internet. The software can be installed locally for private, infinite administration of linked devices and data, but there is also a free tier accessible for connecting a limited number of devices (Figure 9.6).

Any machine with Internet access, including ARM, Sigfox, Raspberry Pi, Lora solutions over gateways, and Arduino devices, to name a few, can be connected to this platform because it is independent of the hardware. Platform includes device registries, bi-directional real time communication for sensing or actuation, data and configuration storage, allowing the storage of time series data, identity and access

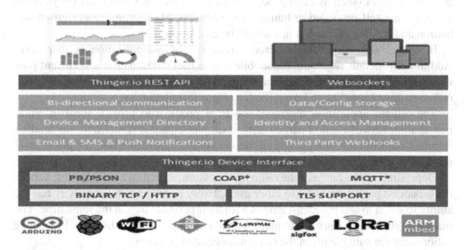

FIGURE 9.6 IoT programs – e Health.

management (IAM), allowing third party entities to access the platform and device resources via REST/Websocket APIs, and third party Webhooks, allowing the devices to quickly call other Web services.

9.5.3 LIBELIUM MYSIGNALS

This serves as a framework for the development of eHealth and medical device applications. The platform can be used to test personal sensors for health applications as well as to develop web apps for eHealth. One commercial product produced and sponsored by a Spanish firm called Libelium9 is MySignals. More than 20 biometric indicators, including blood pressure, oxygen levels in the blood, muscle electromyography signals, glucose levels, galvanic skin reaction, snoring waves, patient posture, ventilation, and body scale characteristics, can be measured using this technology. Sensor data kept in the MySignals cloud or in a third party's cloud so that it can be viewed in other websites and mobile applications. Libelium provides both an open source hardware version (based on Arduino) as well as an application programming interface (API) for access to data by developers. One of the downsides is that the SW version, which runs on the Libelium Atmega 2560 node, is not able to transfer data directly from MySignals to a third-party cloud server; this option is only accessible for the HW version.

9.6 CASE STUDY

Mobile Application: The smartphone application is called SmartGroup@ Net (SGN).

This enables and supports collective outdoor search activities.

The program is beneficial for several government services that may be sponsored when civilian volunteers acting as rescuers use mobile phones. Other potential uses for SGN include enhancing climbing safety, organising and managing rescue efforts in disaster zones (such as earthquakes, aircraft crashes, etc.), and other coordinated actions using self-propelled or human-borne sensors. Maintaining proper group formation and topology is crucial in each of the cases.

In Figure 9.7, an example screen from the SGN application is displayed. Additionally, details regarding the mobile phone user's destination and current position as the locations of more action participants are displayed on the map obtained online or downloaded as an image file for offline installation.

The offered application leverages the BLE protocol to provide local information sharing between action participants. Each participant is responsible for sending information about himself, such as his action number, username, and ID, place, level (regular or emergency), and heart rate.

Depending on the range of the radio transmission, such data are encrypted, kept in the broadcast packet, and sent to other users. Every participant in the activity has the ability to listen to and broadcast emails with their personal data at the same time. The manager (guide) can learn about participants' health position in this way. Preventive actions that are suitable given the circumstances can be taken.

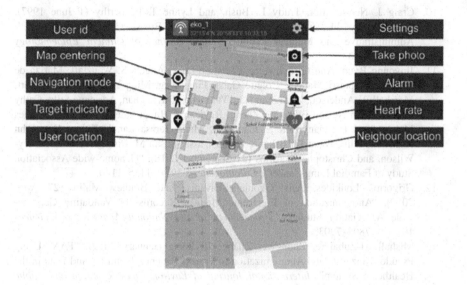

FIGURE 9.7 Instance – SGN user screen (buttons and fields report).

REFERENCES

1. "Personal Health Records" (PDF). CMS. April 2011. Archived from the original (PDF) on 2012-03-05. Retrieved 14 April 2012.
2. Linda M. Spooner and Kiberly A. Pesaturo, "The Medical Record".
3. Jacob Kehinde Opele, Michael Segun Omole, and Tajudeen Temitayo Adebayo (2019). "The Management of Health Records Libraries Through the Lens of Ranganathan's Theory" *Library Philosophy and Practice* (e-journal). 3733.
4. Popoola A. Awogbami, Jacob Kehinde Opele, and Temitope Patricia Awe (2020). "Health Records Management Practices and Patients' Satisfaction in Selected University Medical Centres in South-West", *Global Journal of Social Sciences Studies*, 6(2), 106–114. e-ISSN: 2518-0614.
5. O.A. Bolarinwa, B. Sakyi, B.O. Ahinkorah, K.V. Ajayi, A.-A. Seidu, J.E. Hagan, Jr., and Z.T. Tessema. "Spatial Patterns and Multilevel Analysis of Factors Associated with Antenatal Care Visits in Nigeria: Insight from the 2018 Nigeria Demographic Health Survey". "Medical Records". McKinley Health Center. Retrieved 2012-04-14.
6. Elise McAuley, Chandana Unnithan, F. Soie Karamzalis (2012). "Implementing Scanned Medical Record Systems in Australia: A Structured Case Study on Envisioned Changes to Elective Admissions Process in a Victorian Hospital" *International Journal of E-Adoption*, 4(4), 29–54, October–December 2012.
7. "Medical Records". McKinley Health Center. Retrieved 2012-04-14.
8. S. Nundy et al., How to Practice Academic Medicine and Publish from Developing Countries? 2022.
9. Daniel H. Solomon, Chih-Chin Liu, I.-Hsin Kuo, Agnes Zak, and Seoyoung C. Kim, (1 September 2016). "Effects of Colchicine on Risk of Cardiovascular Events and Mortality Among Patients with Gout: a Cohort Study Using Electronic Medical Records Linked with Medicare Claims". *Annals of the Rheumatic Diseases* 75(9): 1674–1679.

10. Craig J. Newschaffer, Trudy L. Bush, and Lynne T. Penberthy (1 June 1997). "Comorbidity Measurement in Elderly Female Breast Cancer Patients with Administrative and Medical Records Data". *Journal of Clinical Epidemiology* 50(6): 725–733.
11. Jinyoung Byun, Ann G. Schwartz, Christine Lusk, Angela S. Wenzlaff, Mariza de Andrade; Diptasri Mandal, Colette Gaba, Ping Yang, Ming You, Elena Y. Kupert, Marshall W. Anderson, Younghun Han, Yafang Li; David Qian, Adrienne Stilp, Cathy Laurie, Sarah Nelson, Wenying Zheng, Rayjean J. Hung; Valerie Gaborieau, James Mckay, Paul Brennan, Neil E. Caporaso, Maria Teresa Landi, Xifeng Wu, John R. McLaughlin, Yonathan Brhane, Yohan Bossé, Susan M. Pinney, Joan E. Bailey-Wilson, and Christopher I. Amos (21 September 2018). "Genome-wide Association Study of Familial Lung Cancer". *Carcinogenesis* 39(9): 1135–1140.
12. Grigorios Loukides, Aris Gkoulalas-Divanis, and Bradley Malin (27 April 2010). "Anonymization of Electronic Medical Records for Validating Genome-wide Association Studies". *Proceedings of the National Academy of Sciences* 107(17): 7898–7903.
13. Mishall Al-Zubaidie, Zhongwei Zhang, Ji Zhang (January 2019). "PAX: Using Pseudonymization and Anonymization to Protect Patients' Identities and Data in the Healthcare System". *International Journal of Environmental Research and Public Health* 16(9): 1490.
14. Acar Tamersoy, Grigorios Loukides, Mehmet Ercan Nergiz, Yucel Saygin, Bradley Malin (May 2012). "Anonymization of Longitudinal Electronic Medical Records". *IEEE Transactions on Information Technology in Biomedicine* 16(3): 413–423.
15. Raphaël Chevrier, Vasiliki Foufi, Christophe Gaudet-Blavignac, Arnaud Robert, and Christian Lovis (31 May 2019). "Use and Understanding of Anonymization and De-Identification in the Biomedical Literature: Scoping Review". *Journal of Medical Internet Research* 21(5): e13484. doi:10.2196/13484. PMC 6658290. PMID 31152528.
16. Vartika Puri, Shelly Sachdeva, and Parmeet Kaur (1 May 2019). "Privacy Preserving Publication of Relational and Transaction Data: Survey on the Anonymization of Patient Data". *Computer Science Review* 32: 45–61.
17. O. Lincetto, S. Mothebesoane-Anoh, P. Gomez, and S. Munjanja (2006). *Antenatal Care, Opportunities for Africa's Newborns: Practical Data, Policy and Programmatic Support for Newborn Care in Africa*. WHO: Geneva, Switzerland, pp. 55–62.
18. World Health Organization. Maternal Mortality. Fact Sheets. 2019.
19. A.F. Fagbamigbe and E.S. Idemudia (2015). "Barriers to Antenatal Care Use in Nigeria: Evidences from Non-users and Implications for Maternal Health Programming." *BMC Pregnancy Childbirth*, 15, 95.
20. Z.T. Tessema, A.B. Teshale, G.A. Tesema, and K.S. Tamirat (2021). "Determinants of Completing Recommended Antenatal Care Utilization in Sub-Saharan from 2006 to 2018: Evidence from 36 Countries Using Demographic and Health Surveys." *BMC Pregnancy Childbirth*, 21, 192. [CrossRef]
21. World Health Organization (2019). *Maternal Health in Nigeria: Generating Information for Action*. Available online: www.who.int/reproductivehealth/maternal-health-nigeria/en (accessed on 25 June 2021).
22. I. Ajayi and D. Osakinle (2013). "Socio Demographic Factors Determining the Adequacy of Antenatal Care among Pregnant Women Visiting Ekiti State Primary Health Centers." *Online Journal of Health and Allied Sciences* 12, 9152.
23. World Health Organization (2016). *World Health Statistics 2016: Monitoring Health for the SDGs Sustainable Development Goals*. Geneva, Switzerland: WHO.

24. A.F. Fagbamigbe and E.S. Idemudia (2017). "Wealth and Antenatal Care Utilization in Nigeria: Policy Implications." *Health Care Women International* 38, 17–37. 10.1080/07399332.2016.1225743
25. C.O. Nwosu and J.E. Ataguba (2019). "Socioeconomic Inequalities in Maternal Health Service Utilisation: A Case of Antenatal Care in Nigeria Using a Decomposition Approach." *BMC Public Health*, 19, 1493. https://bmcpublichealth.biomedcentral.com/articles/10.1186/s12889-019-7840-8
26. T.K. Tegegne, C. Chojenta, T. Getachew, R. Smith, and D. Loxton (2019). "Antenatal Care Use in Ethiopia: A Spatial and Multilevel Analysis." *BMC Pregnancy Childbirth* 19, 399.
27. Z.T. Tessema, and T.Y. Akalu (2020). "Spatial Pattern and Associated Factors of ANC Visits in Ethiopia: Spatial and Multilevel Modeling of Ethiopian Demographic Health Survey Data." *Advances in Preventive Medicine* 2020, 4676591. [CrossRef]
28. N. Chandhiok, B.S. Dhillon, I. Kambo, and N.C. Saxena (2006). "Determinants of Antenatal Care Utilization in Rural Areas of India: A Cross-sectional Study from 28 Districts (An ICMR Task Force Study)." *Journal of Obstetrics and Gynecology India*, 56, 47–52.
29. L. Omo-Aghoja, O. Aisien, J. Akuse, S. Bergstrom, and F.E. Okonofua (2010). "Maternal Mortality and Emergency Obstetric Care in Benin City, South-south Nigeria." *Journal of Clinical Medicine and Research*, 2, 55–60.
30. M. Dairo and K. Owoyokun (2010). "Factors Affecting the Utilization of Antenatal Care Services in Ibadan, Nigeria." *Benin Journal of Postgraduate Medicine* 12, 1. 10.4314/bjpm.v12i1.63387

10 A Decision-Making System for Clinical Data

Natarajan Rajesh, M. Natesh, Anitha Premkumar, V. Karthik and T. Ramesh

10.1 INTRODUCTION

Cardiovascular disease (CVD) is consistently ranked among the top causes of mortality on a global scale and contributes to around 30% of all global fatalities. The number of fatalities worldwide is expected to rise to roughly 22 million by 2030. A total of 121.5 million persons in the United States have CVD. Nearly half of all fatalities in Korea in 2018 were caused by heart disease, making it one of the most important contributors to death rates throughout the nation. Artery walls in the arteries may lead to a heart attack or stroke if it becomes lodged in the arteries and prevents blood flow. Cardiovascular disease risk factors include a poor diet, insufficient physical activity, and heavy alcohol and tobacco use. Practicing a healthy daily lifestyle, such as cutting down on salt intake, increasing the number of fruits and vegetables you consume, starting an exercise routine, and giving up tobacco are all great places to start. Not drinking alcohol might help lessen the likelihood of developing heart disease by reducing these risk factors. Early identification of cardiac disease in high-risk individuals and better diagnosis via the use of a prediction may result in a reduction in the overall mortality rate, as well as in the ability to make better choices in its prevention and treatment. This has been largely advocated. Incorporating a clinical decision support system (CDSS) prediction model into clinical practice has the potential to improve heart disease risk assessment and drug selection. A large body of evidence suggests that implementing a CDSS has the potential to improve the quality of treatment provided, as well as clinical decision-making and preventative measures. Decision-making based on evidence and clinical experience is a relatively recent notion in healthcare. On the other hand, machine learning is vulnerable to problems associated with outlier and imbalanced data, which can diminish the accuracy of the prediction model. Synthetic minority over-sampling (SMOTE-Out) was discovered in prior research to considerably increase the accuracy of prediction models by rebalancing the distribution of data and integrating a boosted K-means clustering (BKC) based method to detect and remove data that were deemed to be outliers. A combination of BKC, SMOTE-Out, and weighted fuzzy-based recurrent neural network (WFRNN) for cardiovascular disease prediction has not been tested in any previous studies to the best of our knowledge. As a result, we propose a robust heart disease prediction model (HDPM) for a CDSS by combining BKC-based outlier detection and elimination, SMOTE-Out data distribution balancing, and WFRNN cardiac disease prediction. There are three parts to this HDPM. The model was developed by comparing the results of previous research conducted in Cleveland with two publicly available datasets. A Heart Disease CDSS (HDCDSS) has been designed and implemented to test the proposed model's applicability by diagnosing participants based on their present state. Improved heart disease clinical decision-making is envisaged as a result of the HDCDSS created by the researchers. Figure 10.1 shows the benefits of the clinical decision support system. The collection of computer programs that can sift through a patient's electronic health records (EHRs) and pull out the information that doctors need to make a snap clinical judgement.

In most cases, a lack of focus on the part of the doctor was to blame for these kinds of mistakes. Pharmaceutical mistakes may lead to drug interaction, improper dosing, and other inefficiencies; CDSS successfully addresses this problem by automating the whole process. CDSS monitors patient compliance with prescribed therapies and alerts physicians when necessary. Atypical appearances, cognitive mistakes, professional bias, and rare pathological conditions all contribute to a high rate of misdiagnoses. CDSS is quite effective at handling such errors. Clinicians benefit greatly from having everything in one central location. All clinicians may be certain that they are up-to-date thanks to consistent updates and verified data. If the latest medical materials were centralised, duplicative expenditures in various logins for different materials may be avoided.

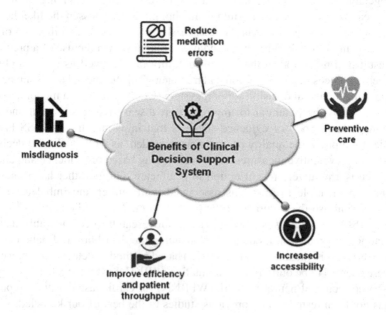

FIGURE 10.1 Benefits of clinical decision support system.

10.1.1 MOTIVATION

Healthcare facilities have significant challenges in providing high-quality treatment at affordable rates. High-quality medical care involves making accurate diagnoses and providing effective treatments. The implications of making poor clinical judgements may be severe, and this must be tolerated. Clinical testing in hospitals must be kept to a minimum as well. The majority of hospitals now employ electronic medical records (EMRs) or other forms of hospital information systems (HISs) to maintain track of patient data. There is a lot of information generated by these systems, in the form of numbers, words, graphs, and pictures. These data are seldom utilised to assist therapeutic decision-making, which is a sad state of affairs. These data provide a plethora of previously undiscovered information. The driving force for this investigation.

10.2 PROBLEM STATEMENT

A large number of hospital information systems are intended to facilitate the billing of patients, inventory management and the creation of basic statistics. Decision support systems are used in certain hospitals, although their scope is somewhat restricted. They can make comments like "Name the unmarried, over-30 cancer patients" Patients' information on cancer treatment options, such as chemotherapy, radiation or a combination, cannot be utilised to answer questions like "Identify preoperative predictors that increase hospital stay" or "Predict the chance of patients getting heart disease based on patient records."

To make clinical decisions, doctors often rely on their subjective judgement instead of the database's richness of data. Biases, mistakes, and unnecessary medical expenses might result from this practice, which negatively impacts patient care. Improvements in healthcare mistakes, patient safety, undesirable practice variation and clinical outcomes may result from combining clinical decision support with electronic health records. Using tools like data mining and other data modelling and analysis techniques, this idea has great promise for creating an environment rich in information that can be used to make better healthcare judgements.

10.3 PROPOSED METHODOLOGY

Figure 10.2 depicts the development process for the proposed methodology. To begin with, data on cardiovascular disease is gathered. In the second step, data preprocessing is completed to be ready for the data transformation and feature selection steps that follow.

In the third stage, we use the optimal parameter to determine the BCK-based outlier identification strategy to find the outlier data. In the final step, outliers are eliminated from the dataset to make it more usable. The SMOTE-out method is utilised to generate evenly distributed training datasets. The next step is to use what we've discovered in the training data to the development of HDPM based on WFRNN and GA. The suggested HDPM is then implemented in the CDSS and its performance is measured using the provided metrics. In order to rule out the possibility of model fitting, we utilised a cross-validation technique. Overfitting in models can be

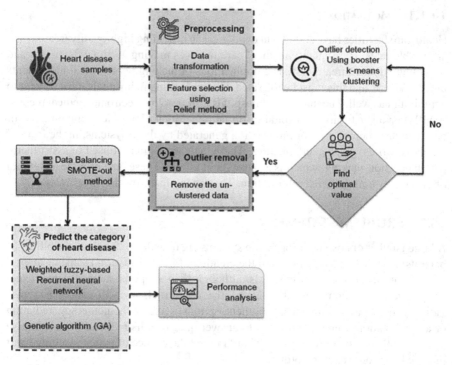

FIGURE 10.2 Proposed methodology.

avoided through the use of cross-iterative validation sampling. Studies have proven that cross-validation prevents overfitting and maintains the generalised model's bias–variance trade-off. The following sections provide extensive detail regarding each step, including descriptions of the datasets and modules employed as well as metrics regarding the stages' respective performance. The results of a comparison between the suggested model and models that already exist are also given. By adding the WFRNN-GA into the CDSS to determine the subject's current heart health, we finally ensure the viability of the suggested model.

10.3.1 Heart Disease Dataset

To investigate the potential of a machine learning model for detecting cardiac illness, researchers looked at the Statlog dataset. After the model has been developed, it will be put through its paces on the dataset to ensure its generalisability and stability. Statlog Heart Disease database at the University of California, Irvine (UCI), has the data set for cardiac research. The initial dataset consisted of 270 people, 13 attributes, and one type of output. There are 120 "positive" for heart disease and 150 "negative" patients. There are no missing values in the dataset. This document provides a comprehensive analysis of the features and distribution of the dataset. The properties of the Statlog dataset are listed in Table 10.1. Statlog dataset mean and "standard deviation (STD)" are displayed in Table 10.2.

A Decision-Making System for Clinical Data

TABLE 10.1
Dataset attributes description for Statlog dataset

Statlog Dataset: Attributes

Description	Type	Date Range
Years of age of the topic	Numeral	[29,77]
Sex of the Subject	Double	1=male
Types of Heart Problems	Minimal	1 = normal angina, 2 = pre pain, 3 = unusual angina, and 4 = symptomatic
Mean diastolic blood pressure at rest (in millimetres of mercury)	Numeral	[94,200]
HDL-Cholesterol (mg/dl)	Numeral	[126,564]
Over 120 mg/dl inside the fasting state	Double	1=true
Electrocardiogram Findings when at Rest	Nominal	0=normal, 1=abnormal ST and T waves, 2=exhibiting signs of or a diagnosis of left ventricular hypertrophy
Vitality level at its peak	Numeral	[71,202]
Inspiring engine via exercise	Double	1=yes
Exertion-induced ST depression compared to resting levels	Numeral	[0,6.2]
The gradient of the ST segment at maximal activity intensity	Minimal	Level = 1, Undulating = 2, and Declining = 3
Colour-coding the size of the vessels from zero to three	Minimal	0-3
Flaw Classification	Minimal	3 for normal, 6 for a permanent flaw, and 7 for a fixable one

10.3.2 Preprocessing

The goals of data preparation are to streamline data, identify relationships within data, standardise data, identify and eliminate outliers and extract data characteristics. Data processing encompasses activities including sorting, organising, transforming and compressing information.

10.3.2.1 Data Transformation

The data processing phase is data transformation, which generally encompasses data generalisation, smoothing, normalisation, and attribute generation. Data normalisation may increase the accuracy and efficiency of data mining systems. If the data has previously been normalised, that is, scaled to a certain range such as [0.0, 1.0], the results are better. Given datasets must be converted to an appropriate data mining format for data transformation to take place. This may be done by normalising or aggregating the data or by smoothing the data. To reduce large amounts of data, one may use several techniques such as dimension reduction and data cube aggregation

TABLE 10.2
Dataset distribution (mean and standard deviation (STD)) for Statlog dataset

No.	Symbol	Present (Positive) Mean±D	Absent (Negative) Mean±D
1	Age	56.54±10	52.70±50
2	Sex	–	–
3	Cp	–	–
4	Trestbps	134.41±.3	128.85±.45
5	Chol	256.47±95	244.21±.01
6	Fbs	–	–
7	Restecg	–	–
8	Thalach	138.85±.10	158.31±.25
9	Exang	–	–
10	old peak	1.58±25	0.62±5
11	Slope	–	–
12	Ca	–	–
13	Thal	–	–

as well as data compression, discretisation, numerosity reduction and idea hierarchy creation to reduce the quantity of data needed.

10.3.2.2 Feature Selection Using a Relief Method

Relief is a selection attribute approach that weights all of the dataset's characteristics equally. Gradual changes to the weights are thus possible. There should be a significant weight assigned to the most critical traits, and a small one assigned to the less important ones. Relief employs RNN-like methods to compute feature weights. The instance for which this value was generated is called R_i. Closest hit H and Closest miss M are two of Relief's closest neighbours. They are both from the same class, thus Relief looks for them both. Using the R_i, M and H values, it modifies the feature A consistency computation W [A]. The performance rating W [A] is diminished if there is a big discrepancy between R_i and H. W [A] is raised, on the other hand, if there is a significant difference between R_i and M for attribute A, which may be utilised to differentiate across classes. m is a variable parameter that may be changed throughout this operation.

10.3.3 Outlier Detection using Boosted K-means Clustering

To counteract data deflection in part due to the disproportion in data partition due to multisampling, BKC employs genetic algorithms (GAs) to pick the initial cluster centre, limit the susceptibility to discrete points and prevent the dissemination of big clusters and so on. The following are the typical stages in the algorithm as suggested:

$$BKC (D, k), D = \{x1, x2,\ldots,xn\}$$

TABLE 10.3
The result of BKC-based outlier detection

Dataset	MinPts	eps	#Outlier Data
Statlog	4.80	9.0	3.0

The smallest possible sum of squares set, k clusters Ci. Algorithm 1 depicts the k-means clustering. BKC-based outlier identification is shown in Table 10.3.

Algorithm 1: Boosted K-means Clustering

Begin
1. *There are several different subsamples $\{D1, D2, ..., Di\}$;*
2. *For n = 1 to i do*

Boosted Genetic K-means(D_n, K'); //executing Genetic K means, producing K' clusters and j groups.

3. *Compute $I_c(n) = \sum_{i=1}^{k'} \sum_{a_j \in C_i} |Z_i|^2$;*
4. *Choose $\min\{I\}$ the refined initial points $Z_i, i \in [1, K']$;*
5. *Genetic K-means(D, K'); //executing K-means genetics redone with a custom beginning yields K'mediods.*
6. *Repeat*

Recalculating the cluster's centroid after merging two nearby ones result of a merger of two distinct locations.
To merge (K' + K) clusters till their total number is k.
End

10.3.4 DATA BALANCING USING SMOT-OUT

With a dense distribution of minority instances, SMOTE may generate useless synthetic examples when applied. The dashed triangle represents the manufactured samples created for applying SMOTE to a minority sample, whereas the cross symbol denotes the minority samples themselves. A difficulty may emerge if two vectors are too near to one other, resulting in an extremely short connecting line. By providing synthetic examples outside of the dashed line, we suggest SMOTE-Out as a solution for dealing with this issue. An example of the SMOTE-Out technique is given in algorithm 2, which also describes the procedure.

Algorithm 2: SMOT-Out

Input: *data u, datataset majority, datasetmajority*
majority, getNrstNeighbor $(u, majority)$ *getNrstNeighbor* $(u, majority)$
$k = size$ $(major\,neighbor)$ $size$ $(major\,neighbor)$
$v = major\,neighbour\,[random\,(1\,to\,k)]$

$$dif1 = u - v.$$

$$u = uPAGEXXX + random(0\ to\ 0.3)\ *dif1$$

$x = (majorneighbour)[random\,(1\,to\,k)]$

$$dif2 = u' - x.$$

$$w = x + randam(0\ to\ 0.5)\ *\ dif2$$

SMOTE-Out takes the majority example that is geographically closest to where it is going off the track to generate synthetic examples in the space of the circle. SMOTE-Out may give rise to an issue about how it prevents overfitting. We approach this problem by drawing the synthetic point from the minority case that is geographically closest to us.

In this case, let's assume that we have a minority example u, and a majority class neighbour, v. For the u–v distance, we may use vector $dif1 = u$–v to obtain the outer vector of that distance. For example, suppose that the outer vector of u, which we'll refer to as v, has an upper bound on the distance between it and the majority class space, which we'll refer to as $(u\ v)$. Mathematically, $u = u + rand\,(0, a)$ dif1 may be used to compute it. To avoid overfitting, we used $a = 0.3$ in this investigation. Next, choose a vector w that is near to u. Once you know the closest minority neighbour of the target, you may use SMOTE to compute the distance between your target and that neighbour. In this research, $dif2 = u\ x$ and $a = 0.5$ are used to compute the vector w using the formula $w = x + rand(0, a)\ dif2$.

Assume that u is the centre of the circle, that the separation among u and x, and that b is the percentage of $dif1$ as described previously. When this is done, the circular area will look like this: (1) The diameter of a circle is the measure of the distance across u and x. (2) The synthetic example will be generated in a circle whose radius is equal to b if an is greater than or equal to 0. Table 10.4 represents SMOTE-Out data balancing results.

10.3.5 Predict the Category of Heart Disease

10.3.5.1 Genetic Algorithm with Weighted Fuzzy-based RNN

First, we fixed the inconsistencies in the trained data so that the HDPM could be learned and generated. LSTM (Long Short-Term Memory), WD-vector document

TABLE 10.4
Outcomes of SMOTE-Out data equalisation

Dataset	SMOT-out (Before)		SMOT-out (After)	
	Minor class %	Major class %	Minor class %	Major class %
Statlog	45.17	54.78	51.76	50.10

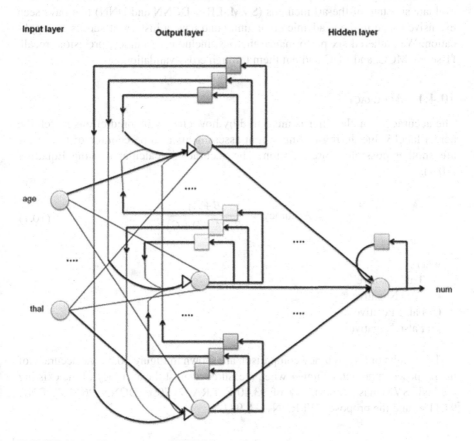

FIGURE 10.3 The structure of W-RNN.

format and NN classification are the three components that make up the W-RNN approach, which was suggested in this research and is shown in Figure 10.3. LSTM is what word2vec uses to get its vocabulary intermediate feature vector (WM-vector). When a text is represented as a WD-vector, it means that the weighted WM-vector was used as the input to the neural net classifier and then was summed to form the vector representing the text. Throughout this study, an RFNN with 13 inputs, 7 neurons in the hidden layer and output layers neurons was used. The weights and biases of the RFNN were each represented by genes that were 64 bits long. A genetic algorithm (GA) was used with a mutation probability of 0.05, a multi-point crossover probability of 0.25 and a population size of 100. The training procedure using GA is shown in Figure 10.4.

10.4 PERFORMANCE ANALYSIS

Results from applying the HDPM to both datasets indicated that it improved prediction accuracy when compared with other methods. For this purpose, we chose to evaluate six state-of-the-art methods (SVM, LRA, DCNN and DNN) that have seen extensive usage in the academic community and have a history of successful application. We gathered six performance metrics, including accuracy, precision, recall, f1-score, MCC, and AUC and put them through cross-validation.

10.4.1 Accuracy

The accuracy of a classifier is measured by how closely its predictions match the actual label value during testing. Right assessments as a percentage of total tests are another possible representation. The accuracy is calculated using Equation (10.1).

$$\text{Accuracy} = \frac{(B+A)}{(B+A+D+C)} \quad (10.1)$$

where
A=True Positive
B=True Negative
C=False Positive
D=False Negative

The results of the accuracy comparison are shown in Figure 10.5. The accuracy of the proposed approach is higher when measured against the accuracy of the existing method. SVM has an accuracy of 93.40%, LRA 95.70%, DCNN 96.80%, DNN 94.11%, and the proposed WFRNN+GA 98.0%.

10.4.2 Precision

One of the most crucial metrics for accuracy is precision, which is calculated as the proportion of properly classified cases to all instances of predictively positive data, as shown in Equation (10.2).

$$\text{Precision} = \frac{A}{A+C} \quad (10.2)$$

A Decision-Making System for Clinical Data

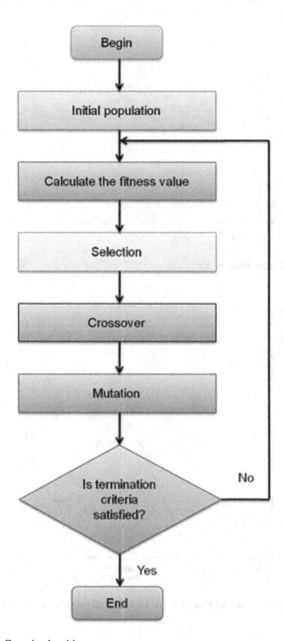

FIGURE 10.4 Genetic algorithm.

Figure 10.6 represents a comparison of precision for existing and proposed methodologies. The earlier methods, such as SVM, LRA, DCNN and DNN, had a precision of 95.11%, 93.21%, 96.70% and 94.15%, respectively. The suggested WFRNN+ GA has a precision of 99.10%.

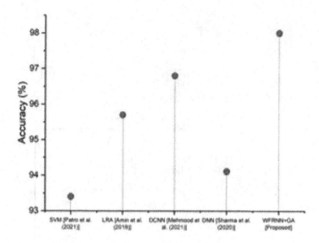

FIGURE 10.5 Comparison of accuracy.

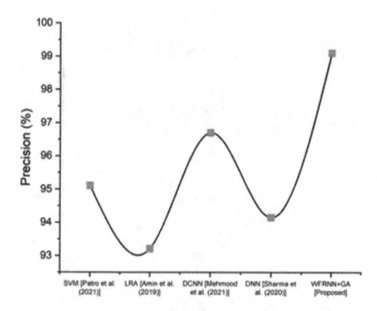

FIGURE 10.6 Comparison of precision for existing and proposed methodologies.

10.4.3 Recall

The percentage of instances that the classifier accurately identified as positive is known as recall, which determines completeness. When a false-negative results in a significant expense. The recall is a performance criterion that helps choose the best model.

A Decision-Making System for Clinical Data

$$\text{Recall} = \frac{A}{A+D} \tag{10.3}$$

The comparison is shown in Figure 10.7, which can be found here. The proposed method exhibits a higher precision level when measured against the existing approach. SVM has a precision of 96.40%, LRA 95.80%, DCNN 97.20%, DNN 93.30% and the proposed WFRNN+GA 99.50%.

10.4.4 F1 Score

The F1 Score is calculated by averaging precision and recall. This calculation determines the percentage of false positives and false negatives. Regardless of how equally distributed your classes are, F1 will often be more useful than accuracy, while being harder to understand.

Figure 10.8 depicts the F1 score for existing and proposed methodologies. The earlier methods, such as SVM, LRA, DCNN and DNN, had the F1 score of 97.80%, 93.15%, 95.18% and 96.50%, respectively. The suggested WFRNN+GA have an F1 score of 99.25%.

10.4.5 Area under the Curve

The area under the curve (AUC) is a statistic that is used to summarise the ROC curve that is used to determine the capacity of a classifier to differentiate between different

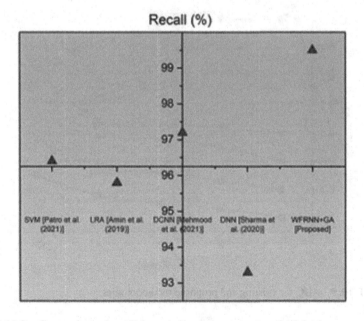

FIGURE 10.7 Comparison of recall for existing and proposed methodologies.

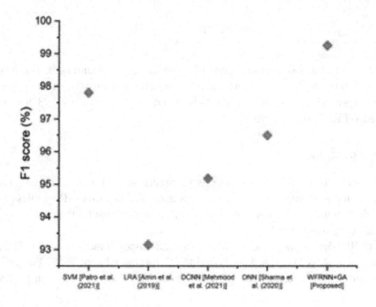

FIGURE 10.8 F1 score for existing and proposed methodologies.

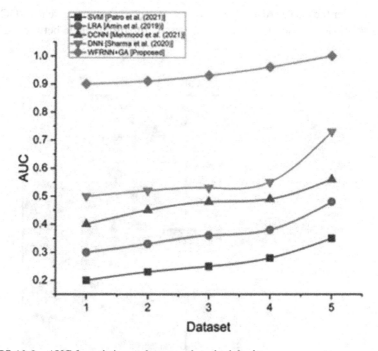

FIGURE 10.9 AUC for existing and proposed methodologies.

A Decision-Making System for Clinical Data

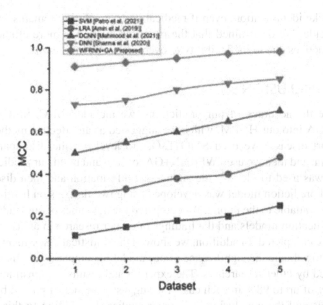

FIGURE 10.10 Comparison of the MCC.

classes. When the AUC value is greater, it indicates that the model is doing better when it comes to differentiating between the positive and negative classifications. Figure 10.9 represents a comparison of the AUC for existing and proposed methodologies. When compared to the existing method the proposed method has a greater AUC. SVM has an AUC of 0.35%, LRA 0.48%, DCNN 0.56%, DNN 0.73% and the proposed WFRNN+GA 1.0%.

10.4.6 MATTHEW'S CORRELATION COEFFICIENT

A statistical technique known as Matthew's correlation coefficient (MCC) is used in the process of model assessment. It is responsible for determining or measuring the degree to which the expected values deviate from the actual values.

Figure 10.10 represents a comparison of MCC. The earlier methods, such as SVM, LRA, DCNN, and DNN, had the MCC of 0.25%, 0.48%, 0.70% and 0.85%, respectively. The suggested WFRNN+GA has a precision of 0.98%.

The parameters show that the proposed method outperforms the existing method, which has several deep issues. These are a few of the issues with the existing strategy. Generally, variables are preferred in the field over support vector machines since the latter requires a lot of memory that is impractical to use with increasingly big data sets. The logistic regression algorithm relies heavily on the assumption of linearity between the dependent variable and the independent variables, which might lead to problematic predictions. DCNN not only shows how well the predictor functions, but also the direction in which the two variables are related. DNNs have shown considerable performance advances that may have a positive impact on clinical practice outcomes like identification, even if medical portrait splitting remains a challenging issue to tackle. We determined that the proposed method is more efficient than the existing practices due to its flexibility to overcome such limitations.

10.5 CONCLUSION

To increase the accuracy of our predictions, we included BKC, SMOTE-Out and WFRNN+GA into our HDPM, which we suggested as an effective method for diagnosing heart disease. We used SMOTE-Out to level out the discrepancies in the training data, and then we used WFRNN+GA to learn and build our prediction model. The BKC was used to identify the anomalous information and then discard it. The generalised prediction model was developed using two datasets on heart disease that were made available to the public. We compared the outcomes of our study to those of other classification models and the findings of earlier research in an assessment analysis that we completed. In addition, we showed the statistical assessment that we had conducted to validate the significance of our model in comparison to the models that were offered by other researchers. The experimental results demonstrated that, with an accuracy of up to 98% in each case, the suggested model surpassed both cutting-edge models and the conclusions of earlier studies. In addition to this, the results of the statistical analysis demonstrated that the suggested model is a considerable improvement over the other models.

In order to accurately and quickly identify the subjects' and patients' heart disease problems, we also constructed and developed the recommended HDPM into the "Heart Disease CDSS." The CDSS collected the patient data together with additional data about the diagnosis, and then it sent all of that information to a protected web server. After that, every piece of sent diagnostic information was filed away in MongoDB, which can efficiently deliver quick responses despite continually expanding amounts of medical data. After that, the suggested HDPM was loaded to make a diagnosis of the patient's present heart disease state, and the results of that diagnosis were eventually communicated back to the diagnosis result interface of the CDSS. As a result, it is anticipated that the created CDSS would assist physicians in diagnosing patients and enhancing the efficacy and efficiency of clinical decision-making about heart disease. To sum up, the thorough CDSS that's been designed and constructed as part of this study is capable of serving as a beneficial guide for health providers.

In future, we are planning to investigate the possibility of contrasting the model hyper-parameters and wider medical datasets with the sampling of other types of data. In addition, more research might be done on a comparison and analysis study using a variety of various outlier identification approaches. Also, as issues of privacy, safety and moment activities continue to develop analysing the possibilities of edge computing and network edge as a way to enhance the "medical decision support system" may be interesting. In the course of our research, we have not yet received any responses from cardiac specialists. In the future, after a particular demographic dataset (from Korea) has been gathered, the opinions of a local heart expert to confirm the dataset and construct a prediction model may be offered. The challenge of the dataset for automatic polyp detection gives us the chance to research cross-data generalisability, which is crucial in the medical field.

BIBLIOGRAPHY

Abdel-Basset, M., Gamal, A., Manogaran, G., Son, L.H. and Long, H.V., 2020. A novel group decision-making model based on neutrosophic sets for heart disease diagnosis. *Multimedia Tools and Applications*, 79(15), pp. 9977–10002.

Adlung, L., Cohen, Y., Mor, U. and Elinav, E., 2021. Machine learning in clinical decision making. Med, 2(6), pp. 642–665. https://doi.org/10.1016/j.medj.2021.04.006

Ali, L., Niamat, A., Khan, J.A., Golilarz, N.A., Xingzhong, X., Noor, A., Nour, R. and Bukhari, S.A.C., 2019. An optimized stacked support vector machines-based expert system for the effective prediction of heart failure. *IEEE Access*, 7, pp. 54007–54014.

Amin, M.S., Chiam, Y.K. and Varathan, K.D., 2019. Identification of significant features and data mining techniques in predicting heart disease. *Telematics and Informatics*, 36, pp. 82–93.

Beinecke, J. and Heider, D., 2021. Gaussian noise up-sampling is better suited than SMOTE and ADASYN for clinical decision-making. *BioData Mining*, 14(1), pp. 1–11.

Blonde, L., Khunti, K., Harris, S.B., Meizinger, C. and Skolnik, N.S., 2018. Interpretation and impact of real-world clinical data for the practicing clinician. *Advances in Therapy*, 35(11), pp. 1763–1774.

Dahiwade, D., Patle, G. and Meshram, E., 2019, March. Designing disease prediction model using machine learning approach. In 2019 3rd International Conference on Computing Methodologies and Communication (ICCMC) (pp. 1211–1215). IEEE.

Dinesh, K.G., Arumugaraj, K., Santhosh, K.D. and Mareeswari, V., 2018, March. Prediction of cardiovascular disease using machine learning algorithms. In 2018 International Conference on Current Trends towards Converging Technologies (ICCTCT) (pp. 1–7). IEEE.

Fitriyani, N.L., Syafrudin, M., Alfian, G. and Rhee, J., 2020. HDPM: an effective heart disease prediction model for a clinical decision support system. *IEEE Access*, 8, pp. 133034–133050.

Freedman, H.G., Williams, H., Miller, M.A., Birtwell, D., Mowery, D.L. and Stoeckert Jr, C.J., 2020. A novel tool for standardizing clinical data in a semantically rich model. *Journal of Biomedical Informatics*, 112, p.100086.

Gárate-Escamila, A.K., El Hassani, A.H. and Andrès, E., 2020. Classification models for heart disease prediction using feature selection and PCA. *Informatics in Medicine Unlocked*, 19, p.100330.

Haq, A.U., Li, J.P., Memon, M.H., Nazir, S. and Sun, R., 2018. A hybrid intelligent system framework for the prediction of heart disease using machine learning algorithms. *Mobile Information Systems*, 2018.

Jefferson, E.R. and Trucco, E., 2019. The challenges of assembling, maintaining, and making available large data sets of clinical data for research. In *Computational Retinal Image Analysis* (pp. 429–444). Academic Press.

Mathan, K., Kumar, P.M., Panchatcharam, P., Manogaran, G. and Varadharajan, R., 2018. A novel Gini index decision tree data mining method with neural network classifiers for prediction of heart disease. *Design Automation for Embedded Systems*, 22(3), pp. 225–242.

Mehmood, A., Iqbal, M., Mehmood, Z., Irtaza, A., Nawaz, M., Nazir, T. and Masood, M., 2021. Prediction of heart disease using deep convolutional neural networks. *Arabian Journal for Science and Engineering*, 46(4), pp. 3409–3422.

Mohan, S., Thirumalai, C. and Srivastava, G., 2019. Effective heart disease prediction using hybrid machine learning techniques. *IEEE Access*, 7, pp. 81542–81554.

Nazari, S., Fallah, M., Kazemipoor, H. and Salehipour, A., 2018. A fuzzy inference-fuzzy analytic hierarchy process-based clinical decision support system for diagnosis of heart diseases. *Expert Systems with Applications*, 95, pp. 261–271.

Ny, L., Rizzo, L.Y., Belgrano, V., Karlsson, J., Jespersen, H., Carstam, L., Bagge, R.O., Nilsson, L.M. and Nilsson, J.A., 2020. Supporting clinical decision-making in advanced melanoma by preclinical testing in personalized immune-humanized xenograft mouse models. *Annals of Oncology*, 31(2), pp. 266–273.

Pandey, A.S. and Singh, P., 2022. A Systematic survey of classification algorithms for cancer detection. *International Journal of Data Informatics and Intelligent Computing*, 1(2), pp. 34–50.

Patro, S.P., Padhy, N. and Chiranjevi, D., 2021. Ambient assisted living predictive model for cardiovascular disease prediction using supervised learning. *Evolutionary Intelligence*, 14(2), pp. 941–969.

Rajesh N., Irudayasamy, A., Mohideen, M.S. and Ranjith, C.P. 2022. Classification of vital genetic syndromes associated with diabetes using ANN-Based CapsNet approach. *International Journal of e-Collaboration* (IJeC), 18(3), 1–18.

Rama, K., Canhão, H., Carvalho, A.M. and Vinga, S., 2019. AliClu – Temporal sequence alignment for clustering longitudinal clinical data. *BMC Medical Informatics and Decision Making*, 19(1), pp. 1–11.

Shankara, C., Hariprasad, S.A., and Gururaj, H.L. (2022). Artifact removal techniques for lung CT images in lung cancer detection. *International Journal of Data Informatics and Intelligent Computing*, 1(1), 21–29.

Sharma, V., Rasool, A. and Hajela, G., 2020, July. Prediction of Heart disease using DNN. In *2020 Second International Conference on Inventive Research in Computing Applications (CIRCA)* (pp. 554–562). IEEE.

Subahi, Ahmad F., Ibrahim Khalaf, O., Alotaibi, Y., Natarajan, R., Mahadev, N. and Ramesh, T. 2022. Modified Self-adaptive Bayesian algorithm for smart heart disease prediction in IoT system. *Sustainability* 14(21): p. 14208.

Tang, R. and Zhang, X., 2020, May. CART decision tree combined with boruta feature selection for medical data classification. In *2020 5th IEEE International Conference on Big Data Analytics (ICBDA)* (pp. 80–84). IEEE.

Uddin, S., Khan, A., Hossain, M.E. and Moni, M.A., 2019. Comparing different supervised machine learning algorithms for disease prediction. *BMC Medical Informatics and Decision Making*, 19(1), pp. 1–16.

Venkatesh, R., Balasubramanian, C. and Kaliappan, M., 2019. Development of big data predictive analytics model for disease prediction using machine learning technique. *Journal of Medical Systems*, 43(8), pp. 1–8.

Zhang, P., White, J., Schmidt, D.C., Lenz, G. and Rosenbloom, S.T., 2018. FHIRChain: applying blockchain to securely and scalably share clinical data. *Computational and Structural Biotechnology Journal*, 16, pp. 267–278.

Zhu, R., Tu, X. and Huang, J., 2020. Using deep learning-based natural language processing techniques for clinical decision-making with EHRs. In *Deep Learning Techniques for Biomedical and Health Informatics* (pp. 257–295). Springer.

Index

A

Absolute Neutrophil Count 245
agility 52, 71
agriculture 121, 185, 187
analytics 4, 51, 53, 56, 58, 60, 62, 83, 84–5, 89, 90, 92, 99, 101, 103
android studio 133–5
aortic valve replacement (AVR) 27
Apache sqoop 81
A priori algorithm 94–5
area under the curve (AUC) 271–3
artificial intelligence 54
Atlas 87

B

Berkeley wavelet transformation (BWT) 211
big data 51, 52, 54, 56, 58, 60, 62, 64–6, 68, 70–2, 75, 77, 79, 81–3, 85–90, 92–103
bioengineering 5
bioinformatics 7
blockchain 13, 87
boosted K-means clustering (BKC) 259
BRATS benchmark 213

C

cardiovascular disease (CVD) 259
Cassandra 82, 83
CCL algorithm 213
Centers for Disease Control (CDC) 112
clinical data 59
clinical decision support system (CDSS) 259–60
cloud computing 14
Cloudera 73, 89
comorbidity 36, 39–46
computed tomographic (CT) 209
convolutional neural network (CNN) 216
CouchDB 88
Ct imaging 20–1

D

daily symptom record (DSR) 251
data mining 58–9, 61, 68, 71–2, 76, 77, 83–4, 91, 93
data warehouse 72
database 59, 67, 70, 77, 81, 86, 88, 92, 95, 99, 100
DCNN 268, 269, 271, 273
decision tree 93–4

deepweeds 122, 125, 126, 185
demographic 109–14
DenseNet 129, 141
diabetes 35–7, 39, 40, 46
disease prediction 121–85
discrete wavelet form (DWT) 211
DNA 58–9, 75–6
Docker 86

E

EHR 8, 24
electrocardiogram 14
electronic data interchange (EDI) 58
electronic health record 36, 46, 243–5
electronic medical records (EMRs) 261
emergency room (ER) 196
endocrinopathies 35
ETL (extract, transform, and load) 68
European medicines agency (EMA) 253

F

FDASIA 9, 30
feature visualization 230, 231
FHIR 10
Flink 73, 85
Food and Drug Administration (FDA) 253

G

GAN 228
genetic algorithms (GAs) 264–5
genome 58–9
genomic data 58–9
Google fusion 89–90
Grad-CAM 229, 232, 234–5
guided backpropagation 229

H

Hadoop 51, 52, 72–4, 80–4, 93
HAN 93, 94
health informatics 1, 2, 4, 10, 23, 29
health information systems 4
healthcare 1–19, 21, 23, 25, 35–9, 46, 52–62, 65, 67, 73, 78, 91, 92, 99, 101–3
heart disease prediction model (HDPM) 250–1
helium drives 75
HGG tumors 216
high-grade gliomas (HGG) 209

Hippa 8–9, 204, 205
Hitech 8–9
Hive 81
hospital information systems (HISs) 261
HPCC 88

I

IDC 18
inceptionnet 131–2
informatics 1–3, 5–7, 9, 11–14, 19, 21–4, 29
information and communication technology 1, 25
in-patient medical records 203
integrated gradients 229
integrated medical record (IMR) 246
International Data Corporation 52
Internet of Things (IoT) 54, 63, 64
IOMT 15

J

JCAHO 8

K

Kaggle 73, 90
K-closest neighbour classifier 111
Kernel SVM 216–17, 220
Knime 83–4
The K-NN classification 216

L

low-grade gliomas (LGG) 209
LRA 269, 271, 273
LSTM (long short-term memory) 266–7

M

MACRA 9
magnetic resonance image (MRI) 209
MapReduce 53, 74, 80, 82, 84, 92, 93, 95–8, 103
Matthew's correlation coefficient (MCC) 273–4
medical data classification (MDC) 252
medical data sciences 35–46
MIPS 9
MobileNet 129–30, 141, 143, 144, 153, 158
MongoDB 72, 73, 75, 81
monitoring system (PRAMS) 112
MRI segmentation 214, 220
MRI 21, 22

N

Naïve Bayes 110, 112
nano instruments 17
nanoparticles 16, 17
NoSQL 52, 58, 72, 75, 81, 82

O

occlusion 227–8

P

Pentaho 88–9
pig 84
Pillcam 17
Plotly 86
PPACA 9
pregnancy risk assessment 112
primary care physician (PCP) 194
privacy 12
problem oriented medical record (POMR) 246
protected health information (PHI) 247

R

R 73, 82, 84, 86
radio frequency (RF) 214
Rainstor 81
random forest classification 212
random forest 111, 112, 117
RapidMiner 84–5
regression 77, 78
ReLU 213
repetition time (TR) 214
ResNet 128, 129, 131, 132
ResNet-50, 128
reverse transcription polymerase chain reaction (RT-PCR) 67
RFNN 267–8
ROC curve 271–2

S

SATMED 18
scalability 71
self-organising feature map (SOFM) 68
sentiment analysis 59
source oriented medical record (SOMR) 246
Spark 52, 72–4, 82
standard deviation (STD) 264
Stats 88
storm 85
structured data 57
support vector machine (SVM) 110, 210
synthetic minority over-sampling (SMOTE-Out), 259

T

T1 contrast enhanced (T1C) 215
Tableau 84, 86, 87
telemedicine 17
TensorFlow 125–126, 134, 185, 188

time to echo (TE) 214
transfer learning optimization 234
tree-based pipeline optimization tool 232

U

University of California, Irvine (UCI) 262
unstructured data 58, 61

V

validity 63
veracity 55, 63, 64, 105

W

Weed 121, 125, 128, 151, 157, 177, 185, 186

weighted fuzzy-based recurrent neural network (WFRNN) 259
WFRNN-GA 262
WM-vector 267
World Health Organization 245, 256

X

Xplenty 87

Y

YOLO algorithm 216, 218

Z

Zoho 87

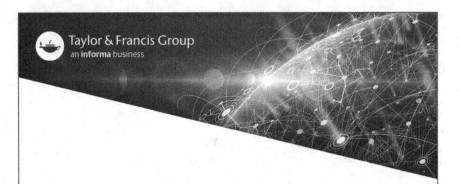

Printed in the United States
by Baker & Taylor Publisher Services